Geyman's most recent book is ¿ medical care is in serious trouble. Tr increased confusion, complexity, and ι ___ ____ _____ expert in what is wrong with contemporary practices. He emphasizes the fraud, waste and abuse in what is only the most despairing of financing that is too costly, care that is too uneven, and financing that leaves high barriers to getting care in deductibles and other patient cost-sharing. No one has monitored this dispiriting development more consistently than John Geyman. He is the most persistent of the many critics of market based thinking and doing in American medical care.

—Theodore Marmor, Ph.D., professor emeritus of public policy and management at Yale University, author of *The Politics of Medicare,* coauthor of *Social Insurance: America's Neglected Heritage and Contested Future,* and member of the National Academy of Medicine

If I could get Members of Congress to read one book this year, it would be this one. Dr. Geyman explains the decisions made by policymakers over the years enabled large corporations to move in and take control of our health care system. I saw this play out during my 20 years as an executive of two of the country's largest health insurers. Those companies and others in health care that are largely beholden to Wall Street have only grown bigger and bolder in recent years. As Dr. Geyman writes, "We can make the case that corruption and fraud are like an undiagnosed cancer defying early diagnosis." This book lays out both the diagnosis and the way forward.

—Wendell Potter President, Business for Medicare for All Founder, Tarbell, and author of *Deadly Spin* and *Nation on the Take*

Medicine for profit instead of public service infects America with rising costs, declining quality of care and worsening inequality of access to healthcare even with the Affordable Care Act. As a prominent medical school professor after a career as a family physician, John Geyman has diagnosed what ails our non-system sick-care system. Geyman also prescribes a cure with lower costs and better care — if we will just follow the doctor's orders.

— David Cay Johnston, author of *The Fine Print: How Big Companies Use "Plain English" to Rob You Blind*

Corporate crime is rampant throughout the American economy, no more so than in health care, where profiteering corruption and fraud are rampant. A single payer system would dramatically reduce corporate crime in health care. A corrupt system of private health insurance would be replaced by a single public payer that would crack down on pharmaceutical and hospital rip offs. In this book, John Geyman gets into the weeds of this vexing problem — and lays out the way forward. As Dr. Geyman puts it — "We have to ask and answer: who is the health system for?" And the answer is — it's for us, not the corporate criminals. This book is an important roadmap to help us crack down on corporate crime and and the resulting violence in healthcare.

—Russell Mokhiber, editor and publisher of
Corporate Crime Reporter, a legal weekly based
in Washington D.C. and the founder of Single Payer Action.

John Geyman has provided an informed and impassioned case for a single-payer system in health care in the U.S. Invaluable reading for anyone who wishes to understand our current predicament or learn what to do about it.

—Kenneth Ludmerer, M.D., internist, medical historian,
and professor of medicine at Washington
University in Saint Louis

Profits, poverty, and politics are a corrosive mix when applied to health care. John Geyman in his latest book reviews the history and dynamics of these factors that cripple modern medical care in the U.S. He is up to the minute, discussing how COVID-19 exacerbates and lays out for all to see the inexcusable failings of our market-oriented method to organize medical care. The reader will find compelling quotes and insights, important facts, and a vision for real change. This is a valuable resource for the healthcare activist.

—Jim G. Kahn, M.D., MPH, emeritus professor in the Institute for
Health Policy Studies at the University of California San Fransisco

How can the United States have the most expensive health care system of all nations yet have it fail miserably in meeting health care goals for so many of us? John Geyman explains the structural defects resulting from a misplaced emphasis on neoliberal policies designed to ensure business successes of the health care/insurance industry when what we need is systemic reform that is designed specifically to ensure affordable and accessible health care for each of us. He shows us the flaws in our system that we need to correct and then provides a pathway for reform.

—Don McCanne, M.D., family physician,
senior health policy fellow and past president of
Physicians for a National Health Program (PNHP)

There is a largely ignored elephant in the room in the national discussion of Medicare for All: the transformation of the American health care system's core mission from the prevention, diagnosis and treatment of illness—and the promotion of healing—to an approach dominated by large, publicly traded corporate entities dedicated to growing profitability and share price, i.e. the business of medicine. That is the underlying pathology in the American health care system that has produced the symptoms of out-of-control costs, declining quality, huge gaps in coverage, and burn out among clinicians. These symptoms have been laid bare by the coronavirus pandemic we are now experiencing.

The corporatization of medical care may be the single most distinguishing characteristic of the modern American health care system and the one that has had the most profound impact on it since the early 1980s. The theology of the market and the strongly held—but mistaken—belief that the problems of American health care can be solved if only the market could be perfected have effectively obstructed the development of a rational, efficient and humane national health care policy. Policies based on this belief have failed.

Dr. Geyman's book persuasively dissects this failure with voluminous and compelling data, presented in an easily understandable form. It's a persuasive indictment of the status-quo, and a convincing argument that our current system must be replaced. Tinkering with it will only serve to kick the can down the road.

—Phillip Caper, M.D., internist with long experience in
health policy since the 1970s, and past chairman of the
National Council on Health Planning and Development

PROFITEERING, CORRUPTION AND FRAUD IN U.S. HEALTHCARE

John Geyman, M.D.

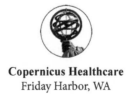

Copernicus Healthcare
Friday Harbor, WA

Profiteering, Corruption and Fraud in U. S. Health Care

John Geyman, M.D.

Copernicus Healthcare
Friday Harbor, WA

Book design, cover and illustrations by W. Bruce Conway
Cover images used under license from Shutterstock adn Alamy
Author photo by Anne Sheridan

softcover: ISBN: 978-1-938218-27-9
Library of Congress Control Number: 2020907318

Copernicus Healthcare
34 Oak Hill Drive
Friday Harbor, WA 98250

www.copernicus-healthcare.org

Dedication

To all Americans who deserve universal access to affordable health care with equity and quality, and have labored under the excesses of a corporatized marketplace that serves the few and ignores the many. And to physicians and other health care professionals having to deal with wasteful bureaucracies of health insurers at the expense of time for direct patient care. May you all see health care reform that ensures care based on medical necessity instead of ability to pay, and returns American medicine to its high standards and traditional ethic of service.

Table of Contents

TABLES AND FIGURES

ACKNOWLEDGMENTS

As with my previous books, I am indebted to many for making this book possible. Thanks are due to many investigative journalists, health professionals, and others for their probing reports on our increasingly dysfunctional health care system. The work of many organizations has been helpful in gathering evidence-based information on what is actually happening at both a macro and micro level as it impacts patients and their families. I have found reports from the Kaiser Family Foundation and its Kaiser Health News especially helpful, together with Dr. Don McCanne's Quote of the Day (don@mccanne.org) that draws widely from so many sources.

Reports from other organizations that have also been helpful include the Center for American Progress, the Centers for Medicare and Medicaid Services, the Center for National Health Program Studies, the Center for Studying Health System Change, the Commonwealth Fund, the Congressional Budget Office, the Economic Policy Institute, the Institute of Medicine (now the National Academy of Medicine), the Lown Institute, the Office of Inspector General, the Organization for Economic Cooperation and Development, the Pew Research Center, Physicians for a National Health Program, Public Citizen's Health Research Group, Single Payer Action, the U. S. Government Accountability Office, and the World Health Organization.

W. Bruce Conway, my colleague at Copernicus Healthcare over many years, has once again done a great job from start to finish of this book, including cover design, interior layout, and conversion to e-book format. Carolyn Acheson has created a useful, reader-friendly index.

Many thanks to my nine colleagues who read advance copies of the book and contributed their generous comments as brief reviews. Most of all, I am grateful to my wife, Emily, for her careful reading and suggestions through many drafts, including editing, proofing, and promotion of the final book.

PREFACE

Health care fraud remains uncontrolled, and mostly invisible. For Americans, this problem represents one of the most massive and persistent fiscal control failures in their history. Many who work the system, or feed off it, like it so. For those who profit from it, health care fraud is not seen as a problem, but as an enormously lucrative enterprise, worth defending vigorously. [1]

—Malcolm Sparrow, leading expert on health care fraud, Professor of the Practice of Public Management at Harvard University, and author of the classic 2000 book, *License to Steal: How Fraud Bleeds America's Health Care System*

Corruption and fraud in U. S. health care have been a problem for many years, mostly under the radar of public awareness and resistant to any effective regulation by government regardless of what political party is in power. The above statement by Dr. Sparrow was made 20 years ago, and the situation has only worsened since then. As a former detective chief inspector with the British Police Service, he knows well about what he speaks.

To give us a launching point to this discussion, here are a few among many examples of health care fraud more than 20 years ago which show that health care fraud was already rampant then:

- Medicare expelled 80 private, for-profit mental health centers from the program after an investigation found that 91 percent of claims were fraudulent. [2]
- Bass Orthopedic, a phantom company consisting of just two rented mailboxes and a phone number, sent phony billings to physicians and hundreds of patients, collecting $2.1 million without providing any services until its bank account was frozen by a federal judge. [3]
- In 2000, Frensenius, as the largest provider of kidney dialysis products and service in the world and with more than 800 dialysis facilities in the U. S., paid a record $486 million as settlements for thousands of false claims and paying kickbacks to physicians for referral of patients. [4]

1

- As the single largest health care provider in the U. S. during the 1990s, Columbia/HCA settled a lawsuit by paying a $1.25 million fine for submitting false claims to a Medicaid managed care program involving falsification of medical records, submission of bills for unnecessary services, including those not ordered by physicians or not even provided. [5]
- Clinical laboratory fraud became a growing problem in the late 1980s. National Health Labs (NHL) settled with the federal government for $111 million for false billings; they had actually altered the forms that physicians used to order blood tests, resulting in their ordering additional tests that sent Medicare's payments soaring from less than $500,000 in 1988 for ferritin tests to more than $31 million in 1990. [6]
- In 1997, SmithKline Beecham Clinical Laboratories, Inc., settled a civil false claims action for $325 million; it had engaged in unbundling laboratory tests, billing for tests not performed, inserting false diagnosis codes to get more reimbursement, double billing, and paying kickbacks to physicians for patient referrals. [7]
- Billing scams became common in the 1990s. Government investigators estimated that fake billings amounted to more than $1 billion by 1998, often involving names of patients and physicians who were unaware of the scheme, with fabrication of entire medical episodes, targeting commercial insurance companies rather than public programs. [8]

Corruption and fraud are arguably much worse today than 20 plus years ago. When we combine Dr. Sparrow's research and warnings with other research findings on fundamental changes in our economy and society over the years, there is no mystery as to how all this has come about.

Matt Stoller, as a writer and Fellow of the Open Markets Institute and former senior policy advisor and budget analyst to the Senate Budget Committee, published an important book in 2019, *Goliath: The 100-Year War between Monopoly and Democracy*. This is his explanation for today's circumstances:

Our systems are operating the way they were designed to. In the 1970s, we decided as a society that it would be a good idea to allow private financiers and monopolists to organize our world. As a result, what is around us is a matrix of monopolies, controlling our lives and manipulating our communities and our politics. This is not just happenstance. It was created. The constructs shaping our world were formed as ideas, put into law, and now they are our economic and social reality. [9]

We can make the case that corruption and fraud are like an undiagnosed cancer defying early diagnosis, such as pancreatic or ovarian cancer, that eats away at the interior of our health care system and evades early recognition and preventive treatments. We have to raise, and answer, who is health care for—the corrupt and fraudulent scammers or patients and their families?

This book has four parts: (1) to bring historical perspective to the changes that have transformed U. S. health care from a mission of service to an unaccountable profit-driven non-system; (2) to describe the adverse impacts of these changes on patients, our population, and taxpayers; (3) to describe and illustrate how corruption and fraud pervade all parts of the medical-industrial complex from hospitals, nursing homes, and hospice to the drug, medical device, and medical information industries; and (4) to ask and try to answer what can be done about all this?

Much of what comes to light here may surprise readers who hope that this problem is not as dire as it is. But you will see that it is. In fact, the current COVID-19 pandemic is exposing the huge shortfalls in our supposedly good health care system, underfunded and neglected public health, increasingly unaffordable care of unacceptable quality, and growing health care disparities and inequities. All that, plus an inadequate federal response to the pandemic.

This will be a rough ride, so buckle up. We need to bring this problem front and center so that we can deal with it in the public interest.

References:

1. Sparrow, MK. *License to Steal: How Fraud Bleeds America's Health Care System.* Boulder, CO. *Westview Press*, 2000, xvii.
2. Pear, R. Cost of rampant mental health care fraud soars in Medicare. *New York Times*, September 30, 1998.
3. Dulbocq, T. Phantom firms bleed Medicare: Cost of fraud in Florida is estimated at $1 billion. *Miami Herald*, August 19, 1994: A1.
4. Kidney dialysis giant guilty of fraud. *Reuters News Service*, January 19, 2000.
5. Columbia/HCA hospital settles Medicaid case of psych care. Report on Medicare Compliance. *Atlantic Information Services, Inc.*, August 12, 1999: p. 4.
6. Sims, C. $111 million payment set for fraud in health claims: Large testing company admits to false billing. (National Health Laboratories, Inc). *New York Times*, December 19, 1992, p. 1.
7. Press release. Clinical laboratory agrees to pay $325 million to settle false Medicare claims. Department of Health and Human Services, Office of Inspector General, Washington, D.C., February 26, 1997.
8. Eichenwald, K. Unwitting doctors and patients exploited in a vast billing fraud. *New York Times*, February 6,1998: A1, C5.
9. Stoller, M. *Goliath: The 100-Year War between Monopoly Power and Democracy.* New York. *Simon & Schuster*, 2019, p. xvii.

PART I

HISTORICAL PERSPECTIVE OF HEALTH CARE SYSTEM CHANGES

Health services may have lingered in the cottage industry stage much longer than manufacturing, but the industrialization and monopolization of health services is now a fact . . . Out of the growing rapport between the delivery and the products industry is emerging a single, American Medical-Industrial Complex. [1]

—Barbara Ehrenreich, journalist and author of *Nickel and Dimed: On (Not) Getting by in America*, and Dr. John Ehrenreich, Professor of Psychology at State University of New York

Writing about his father, Dr. Jonas Salk, inventor of the polio vaccine, Dr. Jonathan Salk, a practicing psychiatrist at the UCLA David Geffen School of Medicine and co-author with him of *The New Reality*, recently shared what he would have expected him to say were he were here during today's COVID-19 pandemic:

If he were here now, he would implore us to remember what made it possible to defeat polio: a national effort to develop and test the vaccine and a world-wide effort to make vaccination available to everyone without profit. Millions donated money and volunteered their children for the largest field trial in public health history. International organizations and governments worked to ensure the entire world could get vaccinated.

My father would insist on also making COVID-19 screening, treatment and vaccination available to all of us, regardless of where we live or our social or economic standing. He would argue that doing so is not only morally right, but profoundly in our national and global interest. When it comes to infectious disease, health—unlike wealth—can't be hoarded by the few. As long as a virus is circulating in an unimmunized population, it's a threat to all, and it's in all of our interests to contain, prevent and eradicate it. [2]

(1) Ehrenreich, B and J. The Medical Industrial Complex. Review of book by Ginzberg, E (with Ostow, M) *Men, Money and Medicine. The New York Review of Books*. New York. Columbia, 1970.
(2) Salk, J. What Jonas Salk would have said about COVID-19. *The Hill*, April 13, 2020.

CHAPTER 1

CORPORATIZATION AND INCREASING PRIVATIZATION: PROMISES VS. REALITY

Control of the U. S. health care system has shifted dramatically over the last 50 years from health professionals and not-for-profit interests to many corporations that are firmly embedded in what has become a medical-industrial complex. That term was coined by John and Barbara Ehrenreich, members of a New York-based Health Policy Advisory Center, in their 1970 book, *The American Health Empire: Power, Profits and Politics.*

What we have today is hardly recognizable from U. S. health care before 1970. Various major elements have led to the medical-industrial complex today, including corporatization, privatization of public programs, a shift to for-profit health care, and closer ties of corporations to Wall Street investors. In this and the following three chapters, we will try to summarize what all of this means.

This chapter has four goals: (1) to describe the growth of health care corporatization in this country; (2) to discuss the extent of privatization of our delivery system; (3) to outline the transformational shift from not-for-profit to for-profit health care; and (4) to compare promises of these changes with what has actually transpired.

I. Increasing Corporatization of Health Care

Before the 1960s, most hospitals and nursing homes were small, individually owned and operated companies. Ironically, the passage of Medicare and Medicaid in 1965 launched the entry of ever-larger investor-owned corporations into the delivery of health care. As these corporate enterprises grew, they typically diversified into other areas of health care with a goal to increase their market share.

By 1984, the 8 largest corporations together owned and operated 426 acute care hospitals, 102 psychiatric hospitals, 272 long-term care facilities, 62 dialysis centers, 89 ambulatory care centers, and a variety of other health care services. [2]

Here is how Paul Starr, Professor of Sociology at Princeton University, described the importance of these developments in his classic, Pulitzer Prize winning 1982 book, *The Social Transformation of American Medicine: The Rise of a Sovereign Profession and the Making of a Vast Industry*:

> *The rise of the corporate ethos in medical care is already one of the most significant consequences of the changing structure of medical care. It permeates voluntary hospitals, government agencies, and academic thought, as well as profit-making medical care organizations. Those who talked about "health care planning" in the 1970s now talk about "health care marketing." Everywhere one sees the growth of a kind of marketing mentality in health care. And, indeed, business school graduates are displacing graduates of public health schools, hospital administrators, and even doctors in the top echelons of medical care organizations. The organizational structure of medicine used to be dominated by the ideals of professionalism and volunteerism, which softened the underlying acquisitive activity. The restraint exercised by those ideals now grows weaker. The "health center" of one era is the "profit center" of the next.* [3]

Matt Stoller described these events in his recent book, *Goliath: The 100-Year War between Monopoly Power and Democracy*:

> *In the 1980s, corporations took advantage of the erosion of merger law by buying their competitors and concentrating industries. Also, a growing number of acquisitions were 'hostile,' meaning the existing management and board did not want to sell the company's independence. [Also in the 1980s] The new rule in corporate America was not to build products or services—it was to buy or be bought. An entire industry of takeover specialists, including arbitrageurs*

who could manipulate stock prices, emerged to restructure corporate America. And this trend began affecting every facet of American culture. Hospitals began a furious merger wave, and costs of American health care began exploding. [4]

II. Increasing Privatization, including of Public Programs

We have had a fierce debate over the concept of universal health insurance versus private insurance and private delivery of health care for more than 60 years in this country. That debate culminated (but by no means stopped!), with the passage of Medicare and Medicaid in 1965. They were both hard-fought by the medical, hospital and insurance industries, but a compromise satisfied the opponents. It was called a "three-layer cake"—Medicare Part A (universal hospital coverage for the elderly), Medicare Part B (voluntary, supplemental physician coverage for the elderly), and Medicaid (an expansion of the Kerr-Mills federal-state program for indigent health care). That approach was intended to limit the further future expansion of social insurance, but that debate, of course, rolls on. [5]

Private insurers have done well since 1965 by being relieved of their worse health risks—the elderly and the poor—allowing them to target younger, healthier, low-risk people. Hospitals and physicians also won by gaining reimbursement for services that previously were not compensated. [6,7] To this day, health insurers, hospitals, and other providers of care in the private sector have pushed for expansion of privatized markets, with subsidies from the government, to meet the needs of the uninsured.

Ironically, most privatized health care has grown up exploiting public programs, first from Medicare, and in more recent years, from Medicaid. In 1982, Congress passed the Tax Equity and Fiscal Responsibility Act, which authorized Medicare to contract with private health maintenance organizations(HMOs) and pay them 95 percent of what traditional Medicare would pay for fee-for-service in beneficiaries' county of residence. Since then, that number has been gamed steadily upward. Figure 1.1 shows how well private health insurers have profited between 2010 and 2016, at taxpayer expense, by revenues from both Medicare and Medicaid. [8]

Did the ACA in 2010 rein in any of this government largess? No way, as CEOs of the largest U. S. health care companies took in almost $10 billion in the first seven years after its passage. [9] This was predicted by Tom Scully, former administrator of CMS in the George W. Bush administration, in these words:

> *Obamacare is not a government takeover of medicine. It is the privatization of health care . . . It is going to make some people very rich.* [10]

FIGURE 1.1

MEDICARE AND MEDICAID KEEP
PRIVATE INSURERS AFLOAT

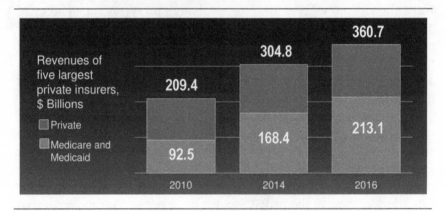

Source: *Health Affairs* 2017; 36:2185

Health care in this country today is dominated by private corporate stakeholders in a medical-industrial complex. Figure 1.2 shows the extent of private ownership in 2016. In effect, we have evolved a system of large corporate welfare for the insurance, hospital, pharmaceutical and other industries that feeds on public programs at taxpayer expense. Administrative and billing arrangements have become very complex, as exemplified by the enormous increase in the numbers of administrators compared to physicians over the last 60 years. (Figure 1.3)

FIGURE 1.2

EXTENT OF FOR-PROFIT OWNERSHIP, 2016

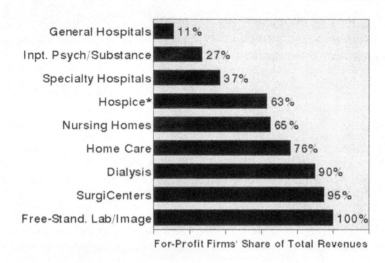

For-Profit Firms' Share of Total Revenues

Source: Commerce Department, Service Annual Survey 2016 *or* most recent available data for share of establishments.

FIGURE 1.3

GROWTH OF PHYSICIANS AND ADMINISTRATORS - 1970-2019

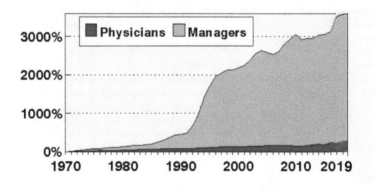

Source: Bureau of Labor Statistics; NCHS; and Himmelstein/Woolhandler analysis of CPS. Note - Managers shown as moving average of current year and 2 previous years

III. Shift to For-Profit Health Care

Predictably, these transformational changes promoted a major shift from not-for-profit care to for-profit care. Table 1.1 shows these distinctions between the two as outlined in 1986 by the Institute of Medicine's Committee on For-Profit Enterprise in Health Care, which issued this prescient warning at that time:

[A substantial increase in the for-profit sector's share of the health care system could]:

1. *Put pressure on hospitals, voluntary organizations, and other facilities that provide needed but less profitable services.*
2. *Create powerful centers of influence to affect public policy.*
3. *Increase the drift of the health care system toward commercialism and away from medicine's service orientation.* [11]

The combination of corporatization and privatization of U.S. health care over the last 40 years, of course, has led to profit maximization and higher prices of care at the expense of patients and taxpayers. Compared to their not-for-profit counterparts, for-profits have higher administrative and overhead costs (especially involved in increasing revenues), much higher compensation of CEOs, and greater likelihood of fraud.

A classic poster boy of CEO fraud is that of Dr. Bill McGuire, pulmonologist turned CEO of United Healthcare. He backdated manipulations of stock options over 15 years and received more than $2 billion in total compensation before being fired in 2006. It finally came to light that he had financial ties to the head of the company's compensation committee, and that the timing of backdating was fraudulent. During his period in office, United Healthcare's stock soared by more than 50-fold, mostly benefitting executives, not patients or health care providers. [12] Many other CEOs were also taking very large stock option packages through various manipulations of their prices and value. [13]

In order to maximize revenue, for-profit facilities such as hospitals and nursing homes typically cut nursing staff, have worse quality of care, and hike their prices. By the late 1990s and early 2000s, there were clear-cut differences in costs and quality of care documented between for-profits and not-for-profits. Investor-owned hospitals, HMOs, mental health centers, nursing homes, and dialysis centers all fit the same pattern—higher costs and worse quality of care. [14]

TABLE 1.1

COMMON DISTINCTIONS BETWEEN FOR-PROFIT AND NOT-FOR-PROFIT ORGANIZATIONS

For-Profit	Not For-Profit
Corporations owned by investors	Corporations without owners or owned by "members"
Can distribute some proportion of profits (net revenues less expenses) to owners	Cannot distribute surplus (net revenues less expenses) to those who control the organization
Pay property, sales, income taxes	Generally exempt from taxes
Sources of capital include: a. Equity capital from investors b. Debt c. Retained earnings (including depreciation and deferred taxes) d. Return-on-equity payments from third-party payers (e.g., Medicare)	Sources of capital include: a. Charitable contributions b. Debt c. Retained earnings (including depreciation) d. Governmental grants
Management ultimately accountable to stockholders	Management accountable to voluntary, often self-perpetuating boards
Purpose: Has legal obligation to enhance the wealth of shareholders within the boundaries of law; does so by providing services	*Purpose:* Has legal obligation to fulfill a stated mission (provide services, teaching, research, etc.); must maintain economic viability to do so
Revenues derived from sale of services	Revenues derived from sale of services and from charitable contributions
Mission: Usually stated in terms of growth, efficiency, and quality	*Mission:* Often stated in terms of charity, quality, and community service, but may also pursue growth
Mission and structure can result in more streamlined decision making and implementation of major decisions	Mission and diverse constituencies often complicate decision making and implementation

Source: Gray, B.E. (Ed.) (1986). *For-profit enterprise in health care: Supplementary statement on for-profit enterprise in health care.* Washington, D.C.: *National Academy Press.* Reprinted with permission

Reacting to the striking ideological gulf between the missions of for-profit and not-for-profit health care, California Representative Pete Stark, as a member of the House Ways and Means health subcommittee, had this to say in 1996:

> *Making fat profits on hospitals at the expense of the poor and the sick may not be a prison offense in this country. What is a crime is the galloping privatization of the nation's health resources and the rise of a competitive health care system that has less and less to do with health and access to care and everything to do with money.* [15]

IV. Promises vs. Realities of These Changes

It has become obvious for a long time that corporate and investor-ownership of health care facilities and services does compromise quality of care and results in worse outcomes for patients, whose welfare should be the consummate goal of our system. We have been sold a bill of goods that the free, unfettered market can bring greater efficiencies and lower costs through competition, but this is patently untrue. Table 1.2 compares privatized Medicare with traditional public Medicare, with the latter persistently winning in every way. [16]

TABLE 1.2

COMPARATIVE FEATURES OF PRIVATIZED AND PUBLIC MEDICARE

PRIVATIZED MEDICARE	ORIGINAL MEDICARE
Experience-rated eligibility	Universal coverage
Managed competition	Social insurance as earned right
Defined contribution	Defined benefits
Segmented risk pool	Broad risk pool
Market pricing to risk	Administered prices
More volatile access & benefits	More reliable access & benefits
Increased cost sharing	Less cost sharing
Less accountability	Potential for more accountability
Less choice of provider & hospital	Full choice of provider & hospital
Less well distributed	Well distributed
Less efficiency, higher overhead	More efficiency, lower overhead

Source: Geyman, JP. *Shredding the Social Contract: The Privatization of Medicare.* Monroe, ME. *Common Courage Press*, 2006, p.206.

Mergers and consolidation since the 1990s have cemented in place the dominant goal of profit-seeking over how to best meet the needs of patients. This has happened despite important warnings in the past. In 1986, the Institute of Medicine voiced a concern that:

> [professional dominance of health care may be replaced by large, politically powerful corporations that] *might "capture" the regulators, molding public policy to their own needs through lobbying, campaign contributions, and use of the media to sway the electorate. . . . The issue, then, is whether it may become necessary in the future to utilize regulation or some other form of societal control to neutralize or minimize the political effects of the economic power wielded by large health care corporations, whether nonprofit or for-profit.* [17]

David Cay Johnston, Pulitzer Prize winning reporter, continued to warn us of the urgent stakes in this corporate transformation in his 2013 book, *The Fine Print: How Big Companies Use "Plain English" to Rob You Blind*:

> *No other modern country gives corporations the unfettered power found in America to gouge customers, shortchange workers and erect barriers to fair play. A big reason is that so little of the news, which informs us about the world around us, addresses the private, government-approved mechanisms by which price gouging is employed to redistribute income upward. When news breaks in one company buying another, the focus is almost always on the bottom line and how shareholders will benefit from higher prices and less competition; much less is said about added costs for customers as competition wanes. This powerful yet subtle bias appeals to advertisers such as mutual funds and other financial services companies who wish to address investors.* [18]

Conclusion

Whether this gaping gulf between corporate-driven health care and the public interest can be narrowed, with a changed goal of service rather than profiteering, will be discussed in Chapter 11. For now, however, we will move in the next three chapters to describe other dimensions of corporate health care.

References:

1. Ehrenreich, B and J. *The Medical-Industrial Complex*. Review of book by Ginzberg, E (with Ostow, M) *Men, Money and Medicine. The New York Review of Books*. New York. Columbia, 1970.
2. Gray, BH (Ed) *For-Profit Enterprise in Health Care*. Washington, D.C. Institute of Medicine. *National Academy Press*, 1986, p. 40.
3. Starr, P. T*he Social Transformation of American Medicine*. New York. *Basic Books*, 1982, p. 448.
4. Stoller, M. *Goliath: The 100-Year War between Monopoly Power and Democracy*. New York. *Simon & Schuster*, 2019, p. 380.
5. Marmor, TR. *The Politics of Medicare*. Second edition, New York. *Aldine De Gruyter*, 2000, p0. 45-57.
6. Gordon, C. *Dead on Arrival: The Politics of Health Care in Twentieth Century America*. Princeton, NJ. *Princeton University Press*, 2003, 25-28.
7. Oberlander, J. *The Political Life of Medicare*. Chicago, IL. T*he University of Chicago Press*, 2003: 108-112.
8. Schoen, C, Collins, SR. The Big Five health insurers' membership and revenue trends: Implications for public policy. *Health Affairs* 36 (2): December, 2017.
9. Siegel, R, Columbus, C. As cost of U. S. health care skyrockets, so does pay of health care CEOs. *NPR*, July 26, 2017.
10. Scully, T. As quoted by Davidson, A. The President wants you to get rich on Obamacare. *New York Times Magazine*, October 13, 2013.
11. Ibid # 2, p. 205.
12. Bandler, J, Forelle, C. Bad options. How giant insurer decided to oust hugely successful CEO. *New York Times*, December 7, 2006: A1.
13. Maremint, M, Forelle, C. Open spigot: Bosses pay. How stock options become part of the problem. *Wall Street Journal*, December 27, 2006: A1.
14. Geyman, JP. *The Corrosion of Medicine: Can the Profession Reclaim Its Moral Legacy?* Monroe, ME. *Common Courage Press*, 2008, p. 37.
15. Ginsberg, C. The patient as profit center: Hospital, Inc. comes to town. *The Nation*, November 18, 1996. p. 22.
16. Geyman, JP. *Shredding the Social Contract: The Privatization of Medicare*. Monroe, ME. *Common Courage Press*, 2006, p. 206.
17. Ibid # 2, p. 246.
18. Johnston, DC. *The Fine Print: How Big Companies Use "Plain English" to Rob You Blind*. New York. *Penguin Group*, 2013, pp. 11-12.

Chapter 2

GROWTH OF MANAGED CARE AND HMOs: HOPES vs. EXPERIENCE

The concept of health maintenance organizations (HMOs) was a radical departure from long-standing approaches to the delivery of health care whereby individual patients accessed care one-by-one through physicians or hospitals. It was promoted by the federal government in the early 1970s as a way to contain health care costs based on the experience since the 1950s of not-for-profit HMOs, such as Kaiser Permanente and Group Health Cooperative of Puget Sound.

The Health Maintenance Organization Act of 1973 was passed by Congress during the Nixon administration. The basic principle of an HMO is a prepaid group practice: "an organized system of care accepts the responsibility to provide or otherwise assure comprehensive care to a defined population for a fixed periodic payment per person or per family." [1]

This chapter has two goals: (1) to review the history of managed care and HMOs in this country; (2) to compare the common practices of for-profit vs. not-for-profit HMOs, including the extent of profiteering and fraud among HMOs

I. Historical Background for Managed Care and HMOs

The movement to HMOs was slow during the 1970s, but accelerated in the 1980s as employees gravitated to what was initially a comprehensive benefits package with lower out-of-pocket costs. [2] HMO growth was further increased as commercial insurers started new HMOs and as many not-for-profit plans converted to for-profit status. Although the HMO Act of 1973 banned explicit underwriting, insurers found many ways to get around that to attract a favorable patient risk mix, launching a debate which has continued to this day over the extent to which for-profit HMOs can "cherry pick" the market. [3]

In their early years, physicians could contract with one or several HMOs. Later years saw tightening of relationships between HMOs and physicians, whereby HMOs took a more active role in authorizing services, deciding on selection and retention of physicians, assessing quality of care, and developing contractual relationships with hospitals, pharmacies, home health agencies, and other provider groups. [4]

The new language of managed care became "covered lives," which became the metric whereby HMOs could track their growth and market shares. Capitation became the method of payment to participating physicians, who were paid a contracted amount each month for each enrollee in their care, regardless of the extent of services provided. That mechanism raised potential conflicts of interest for physicians, who could make more money by providing less care, which HMOs likewise found to their liking. [5]

During the 1980s, when business and government became more concerned with rising costs of health care, they shifted toward capitated health maintenance organizations (HMOs) and selective contracting in order to contain costs, all under the rubric of "managed competition." By the 1990s, business-oriented managers were usurping clinical decision making and professional autonomy of physicians, launching a growing chasm between physicians and insurers as well as tensions between physicians and their patients. For-profit HMOs grew rapidly during the 1990s as larger insurers consolidated, took on selective contracting more aggressively, and soon outnumbered non-profit HMOs.

By the 1990s, some form of managed care had replaced much of the previous cost-based reimbursement and fee-for-service medicine, both for employer-sponsored health insurance and for federally funded public programs.

The term managed care is actually more accurately represented as "managed reimbursement," since care itself is often denied or minimized in order to raise more revenue for the plan. A major landscape change had occurred in U. S. health care, as summarized by the elements in Table 2.1, which show how the business model works. [6]

TABLE 2.1

TYPICAL FEATURES OF MANAGED REIMBURSEMENT

Philosophy	Follow the "80/20" rule
	• Hospitals and specialists account for 80% of total health care costs
	• 80% of costs are generated by only 20% of patients
	• The 20% paid for primary care "gatekeepers" can control the other 80%
Method of payment	Capitation or prospective payment
Impact on physicians	Increasing discounts
	Managed care intrusions, more paperwork and telephone calls
	Increasing workload
	More denial of services
	Saying "no" to patients
	Less choice and autonomy
	Unrelenting regulatory pressure

Source: Adapted from materials developed by Integrated Health Systems, Inc., Arthur Anderson and Company, SC, 1993

By the late 1990s, there was a widespread public backlash to HMOs, blaming them for limiting access to specialists, and intruding on the doctor-patient relationship. [7] The idea of managed competition was being discredited, giving way to unmanaged competition as HMOs began charging more for premiums, offering lower capitation payments to physicians, and easing limits on access to specialists and other services. Not surprisingly, costs again soared upward, and HMOs just passed these costs on to consumers. [8] This led Dr. Paul Elwood, one of the founders of the HMO movement, to conclude:

For those of us who devoted our lives to reshaping the health system trying to make it better for patients, the thing (managed care) has been a profound disappointment. [9]

Ralph Nader went further in calling out the serious downside of this revolution in health care in these words:

> *The HMO and its deepening swamp of commercialism over service, of profiteering over professionalism, of denial or rationing of care where such care is critically needed, of depersonalization of intensely personal kinds of relationships, are all occurring and spreading without sufficient disclosure, accountability and structural responsibility before the damage to life and health is done.* [10]

Despite this temporary setback, however, the private managed care industry moved on. By the early 2000s, a smaller number of larger, mostly for-profit HMOs still covered about 80 million people in the U. S., despite public suspicion about its conflict of interest between making money for their CEOs and shareholders and their responsibility to assure good medical care. Less encumbered by HMO restrictions, a 2001 survey by the Center for Studying Health System Change found that almost 86 percent of responding specialists felt that they had enough clinical autonomy (note that that number is not for primary care physicians!). [11]

Although managed care and HMOs have been disappointing in terms of containing costs system-wide, they have certainly become major revenue centers of a profit-driven system. They have also contributed to a major overall shift from hospitals as the center of gravity to health care systems, with big changes in overall priorities, as shown by Table 2.2. As we shall soon see, however, that doesn't lead to improved quality of care or better outcomes. [12]

II. Common Practices of For-Profit vs. Not-for-Profit HMOs

A majority of HMOs are for-profit as they pursue their mission to "cover the lives" within their defined populations. Some HMOs, such as the iconic Kaiser Permanente program that dates back to World War II years, are considered mostly not-for-profit, but they at times have also, and still do, exhibit predatory behaviors similar to those of their for-profit counterparts. Examples include Kaiser's conduct of a pilot project years ago whereby financial bonuses were given to clerks who spent the least amount of time on the telephone with patients and limited the number of physicians' appointments, [13] and more recently, Kaiser's denial of emergency med-evacuation flights from my home area, San Juan Island in Washington State. Here are some of the ways that for-profit HMOs operate.

TABLE 2.2

TRANSITION FROM HOSPITAL TO HEALTH CARE SYSTEMS

Hospital	Health Care System
Acute patient care →	Continuum of care
Treating illness →	Maintaining/promoting wellness
Caring for individual patients →	Accountable for the health status of defined populations
Commodity product →	Value added services—emphasis on primary care, health promotion, ongoing health management of chronic illness
Market share of admissions →	Covered lives
Fill beds →	Care provided at appropriate level
Manage an organization →	Manage a network of services
Manage a department →	Manage a market
Coordinate services →	Actively manage and improve quality

Source: Reprinted from Shortell, SM, Gillies, RR, Devers, KJ. Reinventing the American Hospital. *Milbank Q.* 1995;73(2):131-160

1. *Cherry pick the market.*

In order to avoid the higher financial risk of providing care for the chronically ill, they can segment local markets by geography and type of employer. [14] Another way is to dis-enroll sicker patients from their rolls, as occurred when one-third of seniors enrolled in Medicare + Choice HMOs were dropped between 1999 and 2003. [15]

2. *Deny services.*

Medical directors of for-profit HMOs are typically expected to deny at least 10 percent of approval requests, and receive bonuses if they exceed that rate. They have several ways to accomplish that goal, such as by medical underwriting to avoid higher-risk patients or groups, revising contract benefits, and setting up procedural barriers for approval. [16] In the early 2000s, Medicaid HMOs in New Jersey were rejecting 17-30 percent of claims for hospital stays, about three times as often as for other managed care plans. [17]

3. *Intrude into physicians' clinical autonomy.*

Physicians' claims of medical necessity are frequently disputed within an HMO, often even by non-physician reviewers, setting up contentious relationships between treating physicians and their overseeing administrators. The goals of each party are quite different—care of the patient in the first instance and cost-containment on the other. Medical directors are often, in effect, practicing medicine without seeing the patient, often across state lines, with just a telephone, rubber stamp and pen. [18] When challenged, as is common, HMOs usually respond by saying they are not practicing medicine, just making coverage decisions.

4. *Undertreatment*

Since HMOs make more money by skimping on care and denial of services, that becomes their business plan. The extent of this problem is more serious than most of us may realize. Today, for one example, almost three-quarters of the 73 million Americans on Medicaid are in private managed care plans, whereby states pay subcontractors monthly fixed amounts for each enrollee. The HHS Office of Inspector General has found that many physicians listed on Medicaid managed care rosters are not available. (Figure 2.2) Medicaid officials have no authority over these subcontractors. The State of California recently found that one Long Beach company had delayed or denied care for at least 1,400 enrollees. [19]

FIGURE 2.2

MEDICAID MANAGED CARE PATIENTS CAN'T GET APPOINTMENTS

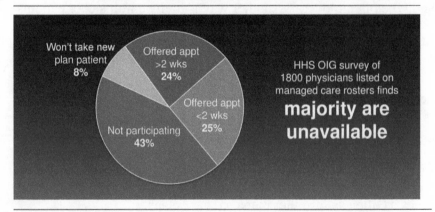

Source: HHS Inspector General's Report. 12/2014 - OEI-02-13-00670

5. *Downgrade quality of care as a priority*

A voluntary national system for reporting quality assurance data was established in the mid-1990s, requiring accredited HMOs to release their performance data to the public. However, compliance has often been incomplete since then. Most HMOs with poor quality of care withhold reporting of their scores. Non-reporters tend to be for-profit and investor-owned, including big names among insurers. Among non-reporters in 1998 and 1999, 60 were Prudential plans, 37 Cigna, 17 United Healthcare, and 14 Humana. [20]

A 1999 study found that investor-owned HMOs scored worse on all 14 quality of care measures than not-for-profit HMOs. [21]

6. *Profiteering and Fraud among HMOs*

Investor-owned HMOs are a big part of a widespread problem of fraud. Much of it is difficult to ferret out from the complex layers of business that separate payers from providers of care and their patients. Whether related to Medicare, Medicaid or other patient populations, there are many ways by which corporate fraud ends up diverting capitation funds from actual care. These are some of them, as brought to light by Malcolm Sparrow in his excellent 2000 book, *License to Steal: How Fraud Bleeds America's Health Care System:*

> "• falsification of new enrollee registrations (either fictitious patients or fictitious enrollments);
> • kickbacks to primary care physicians for referrals of sicker patients to "out-of-network" specialists;
> • fraudulent subcontracts (for example, where no services are provided, or phony management contracts);
> • failing to procure health practitioners so that no service is ultimately provided;
> • retaining exorbitant "administrative fees" and leaving inadequate provision of services;
> • assigning unreasonably high numbers of beneficiaries to providers of service, making adequate service impossible;
> • "bustouts" (money goes in, no money goes out to the vendors, then the entrepreneur claims bankruptcy or simply disappears);
> • withholding or unreasonably delaying payments to subcontractors, providers, or provider networks;
> • destruction of claims;
> • embezzlement of capitation funds paid by the state;

- improper disenrollment practices (deliberately eliminating bad risks—persuading or forcing sicker patients to leave); and
- dis-enrolling beneficiaries prior to hospital treatment (so hospital fees are paid under fee-for-service system), then re-enrolling them once they have recovered." [22]

How can these practices be explained? Here's how Robert Kuttner, co-founder of *The American Prospect*, described this behavior after the "roaring 90s" during the HMOs' heyday:

> *For more than a decade, "market-driven health care" has been advertised as the salvation of the American health care system. In the early 1990s, entrepreneurs succeeded in obtaining the easily available cost savings, at great profit to themselves and their investors. By the late 1990s, however, pressure to protect profit margins had led to such dubious business strategies as the avoidance of sick patients, the excessive micromanagement of physicians, the worsening of staff-to-patient ratios, and the outright denial of care.*
>
> *In an industry driven by investor-owned companies, the original promise of managed care—greater efficiency in the use of available resources and greater integration of preventive and treatment services—has often degenerated into mere avoidance of cost.* [23]

Updating this sorry track record to the present day, these further examples show how little progress has been made to hold private managed care programs accountable:

- Tennessee Medicaid plans, operated by BlueCross BlueShield of Tennessee, United Healthcare and Anthem, have been found to have inadequate physicians' networks, long waits for care, and denials of many treatments, even as the insurers pocket new profits. [24]
- Private Medicaid insurers in Florida have received $26 million over five years for coverage of dead people, mostly as a result of outdated information in state data bases and lack of coordination among different agencies. [25]

- Overpayments to private Medicaid managed care plans are endemic in more than 30 states, often involving unnecessary, duplicative payments to providers and calling for more scrutiny by auditors. [26]
- Centene Corp., the largest private Medicaid insurer in the country, took in $1.1 billion in profits between 2014 and 2016 in California, even as its plans were among the worst performing in the state. [27]

Again, the not-for-profit HMOs, no matter how long they have been around, have at times also joined the gravy train needing more accountability. As one example, Seattle-based Group Health Cooperative of Puget Sound is now dealing with a whistleblower lawsuit filed by a former medical billing manager alleging that it sought to reverse financial losses in 2010 by claiming some patients were sicker than they were, or by billing for medical conditions that patients didn't actually have. Still unsettled, the lawsuit alleges that Group Health retroactively collected an estimated $8 million from Medicare. [28]

Conclusion:

Dr. Paul Elwood, mentioned earlier as a pioneer of the HMO movement, came to profound disappointment in how it had evolved. In the same way, Dr. Robert Gumbiner, another pioneer with 25 years' experience after founding FHP, a staff-model HMO in Southern California in the 1970s, concluded in 1997 that:

> *Today's HMOs, which in many cases own no medical resources but merely contract with physicians and hospitals to provide care, should be regulated as public utilities.* [29]

As HMO abuses have piled up over the years, there have been many attempts at state and national levels, including legislation, to rein in their excesses in the public interest. They have all failed to change their trajectory, and unaccountable profiteering continues on the backs of many millions of Americans.

This chapter, plus the next two to follow, force us to question the ethics of unrestrained markets which continue to violate the public trust. Next, we focus on the growth of investor-owned care, which has become big business and the darling of Wall Street.

References:

1. Somers, AR & Somers, HM. *Health and Health Care: Policies in Perspective.* Germantown, MD. *Aspen Systems Corporation,* 1977, p. 222.
2. Ibid # 1, p. 112.
3. Robinson, JC. *The Corporate Practice of Medicine: Competition and Innovation in Health Care.* Berkeley, CA, *University of California Press,* 1999.
4. Bodenheimer, TS, Grumbach, K. *Understanding Health Policy: A Clinical Approach.* New York. *Lange Medical Books/McGraw Hill,* 2002: pp. 73-75.
5. Ibid # 4, pp. 44-51.
6. Geyman, JP. *Health Care in America: Can Our Ailing System Be Healed?* Boston, MA. *Butterworth Heinemann,* 2002. p. 9.
7. Duff, C. Americans tell government to stay out—except in case of health care. *Wall Street Journal,* June 25, 1998: A 9, A 14.
8. Ibid # 3, p. 62.
9. Phillips, DF. Erecting an ethical framework for managed care. *JAMA:* 280: 2060, 1998.
10. Martinez, B. HMO's grip is easing doctors say, *Wall Street Journal,* January 16, 2003: D4.
11. Nader, R. As quoted in Court, J, Smith, F. *Making a Killing: HMOs and the Threat to Your Health.* Monroe, ME. *Common Courage Press,* 1999, p. 159.
12. Shortell, SM, Gillies, RR, Devers, KJ. Reinventing the American hospital. *Milbank Q* 73 (2): 131-160, 1995.
13. Ornstein, C. Kaiser clerks paid more for helping less. *Los Angeles Times,* May 19, 2002.
14. Robinson, JC. *The Corporate Practice of Medicine: Competition and Innovation in Health Care.* Berkeley, CA. *University of California Press,* 1999.
15. Bodenheimer, TS. The dismal failure of Medicare privatization. Senior Action Network, San Francisco, California.
16. Peeno, L. Approved or denied—how HMOs decide what care you need. *U. S. News and World Report* 124 (9), March 9, 1998.
17. Freudenheim, M. Some concerns thrive on Medicaid patients. *New York Times,* February 19, 2003: C1.
18. Peeno, L. A physician answers questions about denial of care in managed care corporations. *Citizen Action,* 1996.
19. Terhune, C. Coverage denied Medicaid patients suffer as layers of private companies profit. *Kaiser Health News,* January 3, 2019.
20. Press release. Quality reporting dropouts in 1998 and 1999. Physicians for a National Health Program, September 20, 2002.
21. Himmelstein, DU, Woolhandler, S. Hellander, I et al. Quality of care in investor-owned vs not-for-profit HMOs. *JAMA* 282, 1999.

22. Sparrow, MK. *License to Steal: How Fraud Bleeds America's Health Care System*. Boulder, CO. *Westview Press*, 71, 106-107, 2000.
23. Kuttner, R. The American health care system: Wall Street and health care. *N Engl J Med* 340: 664-668, 1999.
24. Himmelstein, DU. Woolhandler, S. The post-launch problem: the Affordable Care Act's persistently high administrative costs. *Health Affairs Blog*, May 27, 2015.
25. Chang, D. Florida paid Medicaid insurers $26 million to cover dead people, report says. *Miami Herald*, December 13, 2016.
26. Herman, B. Medicaid's unmanaged care. *Modern Healthcare*, April 30, 2016.
27. Terhune, C, Gorman, A. Enriched by the poor: California's health insurers make billions through Medicaid. *Kaiser Health News*, November 6, 2017.
28. Schulte, F. Whistleblower alleges Medicare fraud at iconic Seattle-based health plan. *Kaiser Health News*, October 18, 2019.
29. Gumbiner, R. FHP: The evolution of a managed care health maintenance organization, 1993-1997, Volume II. Berkeley: *University of California Press*, 1997.

Chapter 3

GROWTH IN INVESTOR-OWNED HEALTH CARE: FREE MARKETS TO THE RESCUE?!

As we have seen in earlier chapters, U. S. health care has undergone a massive transformation from a largely person-based cottage industry to today's enormous medical-industrial complex, built for the purposes of making money, not service to patients. Here we will try to better understand these changes, with three goals: (1) to briefly discuss the claimed advantages of a free market approach to the delivery of health care in this country; (2) to describe where our largely privatized, corporate market-based system has taken us; and (3) to consider how the deregulated free market in health care has failed the common good.

I. The Persistent, Questionable Rationale for Free Market Competition

Advocates of free markets in health care have held sway over health policy in this country for some four decades. They keep telling us that the competitive marketplace will bring lower costs, more efficiency, less waste, and improved quality of care. Conservative think tanks have broadcast this message since the 1980s through a wide range of media. Here is one such example of market ideology in health care as put forth by senior fellows at the Hoover Institution in 2006:

> *Greater reliance on individual choice and free markets are the solutions to what ails our health care system—a handful of policy changes that harness the power of markets for health services have the potential to give patients and their physicians more control over health-care choices, create more health insurance options, lower health costs, reduce the number of uninsured persons—and give workers a pay increase to boot.* [1]

The dirty little secret is that these promises have been disproven by experience for many years, and have been rebutted elsewhere. [2] Nevertheless, the corporate train has rolled on, even picking up speed. Matt Stoller, whom we met earlier, wrote about this fundamental change in his 2019 book, *Goliath: The 100 Year War between Monopoly Power and Democracy*:

> *By the end of the 1980s, Wall Street had permanently changed corporate America. A new type of business model existed. The leveraged buyout industry, stung with bad publicity, rebranded as "private equity." While some PE firms made productive investments, they were largely tools of floating capital that sought to use the corporation for the purpose of the financier.*
>
> *Strategically, the only businesses that were sustainable in the new legal environment were those that could withstand the pressures of financial raiders. Large-scale monopolistic corporations such as General Electric and Walmart could use the new tools to their advantage. So could high-tech concerns such as Microsoft that had taken advantage of the technology revolution to acquire choke holds over new vital arteries of commerce. Private equity firms and financial intermediaries who could use the new capital market structure to their advantage increasingly controlled American business* [3]

The belief that "competition" lowers costs, as proclaimed by proponents of the free marketplace in health care, is a myth. The track record over many years with higher prices and costs makes that clear. Our increasingly corporatized and consolidated for-profit delivery system is bent on maximizing profits instead of lowering costs in a more efficient system.

The non-profit Center for Studying Health System Change has long studied this issue. It conducted a nine-year study of 12 major health care markets in its Community Tracking Study involving 60 communities, 60,000 households and 12,000 physicians. It found four major barriers to efficiency: (1) providers' market power; (2) absence of potentially efficient provider systems; (3) employers' inability to push the system toward efficiency and quality; and (4) insufficient health plan competition. In 2004, it concluded that there is insufficient competition among local health care systems, and that providers have enough market power to dictate the terms of their arrangements with insurers. [4]

The idea that patients can shop for their best options of care, as they can when buying a car or in other markets, is put to rest when we consider that patients often don't know their actual needs, when urgency of time is frequently a controlling factor, information is usually not available about costs and prices, and consolidation of corporate providers tends to restrict their choices. It is now well known that, as hospital systems gain market share in their areas, their prices and costs go up, as do the costs of medical outpatient services as hospitals buy up more physician groups. [5]

II. Where Has the Corporatized Marketplace Taken Us?

That health care has become big business for corporate America, shareholders and investors has become obvious from an early 2020 article in *Modern Healthcare* reporting that the 2018 revenue ($913 billion) for the seven largest U. S. publicly traded health insurers is approaching $1 trillion. Their profits increased by a combined 66 percent in 2019, driven by massive mergers and acquisitions in 2018. Their combined membership now covers 165 million enrollees, one-half of the U. S. population. The Big 7 insurers —Anthem, Centene Corp., Cigna, CVS Health, Humana, Molina Healthcare and United Health— are starting to see themselves as "health service companies" as they acquire other businesses, such as pharmacies and pharmacy benefit managers. [6]

Here are three ways that reveal how these developments lay bare the extent to which corporate stakeholders in market-based medicine are running roughshod over the needs of patients and their families.

1. Growth of corporate investor-owned chains

Since the 1980s, investor-owned chains have grown across most parts of the medical-industrial complex, ranging from acute care and rehabilitation hospitals to psychiatric hospitals and nursing homes. In every case, by pursuing the business model, the primary mission is to gain market share and increase revenue, not patient care.

Expansion of these chains into related areas is commonplace. In order to increase their market share, as one example, investor-owned hospital chains adopt such strategies as establishing urgent-care clinics, freestanding "emergicenters," and other patient feeder systems. [7] They also tend to locate in more profitable markets and avoid "poor pay" patients, leaving their care to public and not-for-profit hospitals. [8]

These changes upset earlier relationships among physicians, hospitals, HMOs, and insurers. Some non-profit hospitals converted to for-profit status, many by being acquired by investor-owned chains, while others were forced to close. Hospitals had to negotiate contracts with HMOs for sources of patients. Physicians in the community may have contracts with more than one HMO, thereby dividing their loyalty to any one hospital. [9] Charity care went down as HMO penetration in an area grew, while some HMOs even forbid physicians from seeing non-paying patients. [10]

Today, as hospital systems buy up physicians' practices, almost two-thirds of U. S. physicians are employed by them. These physicians are often hired under productivity-based contracts that reward them for providing a higher volume of services and ordering more expensive tests. [11] Not surprisingly, a 2014 study documented that hospital ownership of physicians' practices drives up prices and costs. [12]

Some of the largest health insurers are now breaking up previous relationships with both hospitals and physicians. This has brought new worries to rival physician groups and hospital companies that have invested deeply in buying up physician practices, who now find themselves competing against offerings of insurers. Insurer plans built around its own clinics usually include smaller networks with more limited choice of physicians and hospitals. That can lower premiums and retain revenue within insurers' holdings, but lead to increased costs for patients later when they need out-of-network care. Hospitals are concerned that primary care physicians employed by these new rival insurer competitors will refer patients elsewhere for imaging, other procedures, specialist and hospital care. [13]

2. Poor quality of care in investor-owned for-profit care vs not-for-profits

Many studies have documented that investor-owned facilities and services have higher costs and lower quality compared with their not-for-profit counterparts. Table 3.1 shows the breadth and consistency of these findings. [14-24]

Table 3.1

INVESTOR-OWNED CARE vs. NOT-FOR-PROFIT CARE

COMPARATIVE EXAMPLES

Hospitals	Higher costs, fewer nurses, and higher death rates [14,15]
Emergency medical services	Higher prices, worse care with slower response times. [16]
HMOs	Worse scores on all 14 quality of care measures. [17]
Nursing homes	Often in corporate chains, have lower staffing levels, worse quality of care, and higher death rates. [18]
Mental health centers	Restrictive barriers and limits to care, such as premature discharge without adequate outpatient care. [19]
Dialysis centers	Mortality rates 19 to 24 percent higher;[20] 53 percent less likely to be put on a transplant waiting list. [21]
Assisted living facilities	Many critical incidents of physical, emotional, or sexual abuse of patients. [22]
Home health agencies	Higher costs, lower quality of care. [23]
Hospice	Missed visits and neglect of patients dying at home. [24]

These predictable results of the long-held meme that corporations can help us through "competition and efficiency" of an unfettered marketplace comes as no surprise to George Annas, J.D., leading bioethicist and Professor of Law at Boston University, who saw this coming more than 20 years ago:

The market metaphor leads us to think about medicine in already-familiar ways: emphasis is placed on efficiency, profit maximization, customer satisfaction, ability to pay, planning, entrepreneurship, and competitive models. The ideology of medicine is displaced by the ideology of the marketplace. Trust is replaced with caveat emptor. There is no place for the poor and uninsured in the market model. Business ethics supplant medical ethics as the practice of medicine becomes corporatized. Hospitals become cost centers. Nonprofit medical organizations tend to be corrupted by adopting the values of their for-profit competitors. A management degree becomes as important as a medical degree. Public institutions, by definition, cannot compete in the for-profit arena, and risk demise, second-class status, or privatization. [25]

3. Investor-owned corruption and fraud

Along the way in their business dealings, the lines between corrupt intent and fraud are frequently blurred, especially when private equity firms are involved. This is how they often work when it comes to expansion of hospital systems:

Typically, [private equity] firms begin by acquiring a small hospital system, referred to as a platform company, in a leveraged buyout. Then they add smaller hospitals in geographically disbursed regions, creating a national, multi-state hospital chain. The purchases are all financed with borrowed money, and the private equity firms transfer the debt load onto the hospitals . . . The private equity owners plan to exit investments they acquire in three to five years. . .

These acquisitions usually fall below the deal size that triggers review by antitrust regulators, allowing them to go unchallenged. [26]

Here is another example involving investor-owned nursing home chains. The Carlyle Group, one of the richest private equity firms in the world, made a mockery of "serving" the nation's poorest and most vulnerable people by buying, and then neglecting Manor Care, the second largest nursing home chain in the country. Hundreds of layoffs were announced, soon after this acquisition, staffing was inadequate, and the predictable results were growing numbers of serious health-code violations and harm to patients. The company finally filed for bankruptcy, but only after investors had taken $1.3 billion from it. [27]

III. How Free Markets Fail the Common Good in Health Care

The U. S. experiment with market-based medicine over the last 40 years has failed the public interest. When we look at the totally unacceptable results of quality studies shown in Table 3.1, how can we possibly conclude that this is, or should be, a new normal?

We are way off the track. With the federal government's Strategic National Stockpile nearly emptied out for essential supplies to deal with the COVID-19 pandemic, and with states bidding against each other to get them, prices have gone through the roof—N95 masks went up by more than 1,500 percent (from $0.38 to $5.75!). [28] Medical billing fraud, ironically enabled by electronic medical records, is now costing patients and taxpayers about $270 billion a year (10 percent of all health care costs!) Isn't it way past time to hold the privatized market more accountable?

These three observations—current, 1999 and some 250 years ago—serve to remind ourselves that health care reform is finally an urgent priority.

We have to remind everyone who has entered our healthcare system in the past quarter of a century for profit rather than patients that "affordable, patient-centered, evidence-based care" is more than a marketing pitch or a campaign.

It is our health, the future of our children and our nation. High-priced healthcare is America's sickness and we are all paying, being robbed. When the medical industry presents us with the false choice of your money or your life, it's time for all of us to take a stand for the latter. [29]

—Dr. Elizabeth Rosenthal, emergency physician and author of the excellent 2017 book, *An American Sickness: How Healthcare Became Big Business and How You Can Take It Back.*

Our main objection to investor-owned care is not that it wastes taxpayers' money, not even that it causes modest decrements in quality.

The most serious problem with such care is that it embodies a new value system that severs the communal roots and samaritan traditions of hospitals, makes doctors and nurses the instruments of investors, and views patients as commodities. In nonprofit settings, avarice vies with beneficence for the soul of medicine; investor ownership marks the triumph of greed. A fiscal conundrum constrains altruism on the part of nonprofit hospitals: No money no mission. With for-profit hospitals, the money is the mission; form follows profit—health care is too precious, too intimate, and corruptible to entrust to the market. [30]

—David Himmelstein, M.D. and Steffie Woolhandler, M.D., general internists, health policy experts and distinguished professors of public health at the City University of New York.

And finally:

Government is instituted for the common good: for the protection, safety, prosperity, and happiness for the people; and not for the profit, honor, or private interest of any one man, family, or class of men. [31]

—John Adams, second U. S. president and one of our founding fathers

Conclusion

Deregulation and Wall Street can never serve the public interest. Isn't a 40-year track record enough to prove that?! Remarkably, despite its poor track record, investor-owned health care still reigns supreme over our market-based system, with these long-standing questions still unanswered:

- Is health care a basic human need and right, or is it just another commodity for sale on the open market?
- Whom should the health care system serve primarily, the patient or the corporate stakeholders in providing care?
- Should the delivery of health care be based on the market system or on a public utility model?
- If the private market is to retain its central role in U. S. health care, can its excesses be regulated in the public interest?

We will try to deal with these questions in the final two chapters, but for now, we turn to the next chapter to consider how the ethical basis for health care has devolved as the medical-industrial complex has taken over our system.

References:

1. Cogan, JF, Hubbard, RG, Kessler, DP. Keep government out. *Wall Street Journal*, January 13, 2006: A12.
2. Geyman, JP. Myths and memes about single-payer health insurance in the United States: A rebuttal to conservative claims. *Int J Health Serv* 35 (1): 63-90, 2005.
3. Stoller, M. *Goliath: The 100 Year War between Monopoly Power and Democracy*. New York. *Simon & Schuster*, 2019, p. 405.
4. Nichols, LM et al. Are market forces strong enough to deliver efficient health care systems? Confidence is waning. *Health Affairs* 23 (2): 8-21, 2004.
5. Neprash, HT, Chernew, ME, Hicks AL et al. Association of financial integration with commercial health care prices. *JAMA Internal Medicine*, October 19, 2015.
6. Livingston, S. Publicly traded health insurers' revenue nears $1 trillion mark. *Modern Healthcare*, February 20, 2020.
7. Lindorff, D. *Marketplace Medicine: The Rise of the For-Profit Hospital Chains*. New York. *Bantam Books*, 1992, p. 276.
8. Martinez, B. After an era of dominant HMOs, hospitals are turning the tables. *Wall Street Journal Online*, April 12, 2002.
9. Freudenheim, M, Abelson, R. HealthSouth regroups in effort to avoid bankruptcy. *New York Times*, March 21, 2003.
10. Himmelstein, DU, Woolhandler, S, Hellander, I. *Bleeding the Patient: The Consequences of Corporate Health Care*. Monroe, ME. *Common Courage Press*, 2003, p. 77.

11. O'Malley, AS, Bond AM, Berenson, RA. *Rising hospital employment of physicians: Better quality, higher costs?* Washington, D.C. Center for Studying Health System Change. Issue Brief No. 136, August, 2011.

12. Baker, LC, Bundorf, MK, Kessler, DP. Vertical integration: hospital ownership of physicians' practices is associated with higher prices and spending. *Health Affairs* 36: 756-763, 2014.

13. Mathews, AW. Physicians, hospitals meet their new competitor: insurer-owned clinics. *Wall Street Journal*, February 23, 2020.

14. Silverman, EM et al. The association between for-profit hospital ownership and increased Medicare spending. *N Engl J Med* 341: 420, 1999.

15. Yuan, Z. The association between hospital type and mortality and length of stay: A study of 16.9 million hospitalized Medicare beneficiaries. *Med Care* 38: 231, 2000.

16. Ivory, D, Protess, B, Daniel, J. When you dial 911 and Wall Street answers. *New York Times*, June 25, 2016.

17. Himmelstein, DU et al. Quality of care in investor-owned vs. not-for-profit HMOs. *JAMA* 282: 159, 1999.

18. Whoriskey, P. Keating, D. Overdoses, bedsores, broken bones: What happened when a private-equity firm sought to care for society's most vulnerable? *The Washington Post,* November 25, 2018.

19. Munoz, R. How health care insurers avoid treating mental illness. *San Diego Union Tribune*, May 22, 2002.

20. Devereaux, PJ et al. Comparison of mortality between private for-profit and private not-for-profit hemodialysis centers: A systematic review and meta-analysis. *JAMA* 288: 2449: 2002.

21. Garg, RP et al. Effect of the ownership of dialysis facilities and patients' survival and referral for transplantation. *N Engl J Med* 341: 1653, 1999.

22. Pear, R. U. S. pays billions for 'assisted living,' but what does it get? *New York Times*, February 13, 2018.

23. Cabin, W, Himmelstein, DU, Siman, ML et al. For-profit Medicare home health agencies' costs appear higher and quality appears lower compared to not-for-profit agencies. *Health Affairs* 33 (8): 1460-1465, 2014.

24. Waldman, P. Preparing Americans for death lets hospices neglect end of life. *Bloomberg*, July 22, 2011.

25. Annas, GL. *Some Choice: Law, Medicine and the Market.* New York. *Oxford University Press*, 1998: p. 46.

26. Appelbaum, E. *How private equity makes you sicker. The American Prospect,* Fall 2019, 62-65.

27. Buchheit, P. Private health care is an act of terrorism. *Common Dreams*, July 20, 2015, p. 1.

28. Diaz, D, Sands, G,Alesci, C. Protective equipment costs increase over 1000% amid competition and surge in demand. *CNN Politics*, April 16, 2020

29. Rosenthal, E. *An American Sickness: How Healthcare Became Big Business and How You Can Take It Back.* New York. *Penguin Press,* 2017, p. 330.

30. Woolhandler, S, Himmelstein, DU. When money is the mission—The high costs of investor-owned care. *N Engl J Med* 341: 444-446, 1999.

31. Adams, as quoted by Hartmann, T. A red privatization story. *The Progressive Populist*, November 15, 2011, p. 11.

Chapter 4

CHANGING ETHICS WITHIN THE MEDICAL-INDUSTRIAL COMPLEX: FROM SERVICE TO GREED

The essence of medicine is so different from that of ordinary business that they are inherently at odds. Business concepts of good management may be useful in medical practice, but only to a degree. The fundamental ethos of medical practice contrasts sharply with ordinary commerce, and market principles do not apply to the relationship between physician and patient. Such insights have not stopped the advance of the medical-industrial complex, or prevented the growing domination of market ideology over medical professionalism. [1]

—Dr. Arnold Relman, internist, former
editor of the *New England Journal of Medicine*, and critical
observer of the medical-industrial complex

It is difficult to overstate the significance of the ideas that Milton Friedman launched in 1970, now compounded by the Citizens United decision and the power granted to make corporate values, already dominant, pervasive in every aspect of American life . . . Citizens United is to the expansion of corporate power what the big bang was to the beginning of the universe. [2]

—David C. Johnston, Pulitzer Prize winning investigative
reporter and author of *The Fine Print: How Big
Companies Use "Plain English" to Rob You Blind*

The above two observations illustrate well the polar opposites in mission and values of what has become health care in America. Because the gulf between them is so wide, we have to expect tensions and disputes at the core of what we call a health care system.

This chapter tries to make some sense of these differences, with three goals: (1) to trace some major landmark changes over the last 50-plus years that have produced today's corporatized health care system that places profits above patients; (2) to give examples of how the "invisible hand" of the marketplace and its business "ethic" have corrupted long-standing health care traditions of service; and (3) to consider whether conservatives and business interests can *ever* join in support of providing universal access to necessary health care of our population.

I. Historical Perspective

The early story of health insurance gives us an interesting backdrop to the later medical industrial complex and corporatization of U. S. health care. The original idea for prepaid health insurance in this country dates back to a 1932 report by the Committee on the Costs of Medical Care (CCMC), which made these recommendations that are still relevant today:

1. *Medical service should be furnished largely by organized groups.*
2. *Basic public health services should be extended so they will be available to the entire population according to its needs.*
3. *The costs of medical care should be placed on a group payment basis through the use of insurance or taxation or both.* [3]

Blue Cross originated in late 1929 in Dallas, Texas when the Baylor University Hospital agreed to provide 1,500 school teachers up to 21 days of hospital care a year for $6.00 a person. [4] Baylor soon extended this arrangement to several thousand people in other groups, and the race to provide this kind of insurance was on. Blue Cross and Blue Shield established their first private health insurance plans on a nonprofit basis, whereby more people could afford care, with minimal out-of-pocket payments, and hospital beds could be kept open. [5]

The first warning call about a growing medical-industrial complex as a threat to traditional ethics and relationships between physicians and patients was issued by John and Barbara Ehrenreich in their 1970 book, *The American Health Empire: Power, Profits and Politics.* As members of the New York-based Health Policy Advisory Center (Health PAC), they called attention to these major system changes after World War II in the U. S.: growth of technology and its products, the replacement of physicians by hospitals at the center of a new system, the growing shift to institutionalized medicine, and ways in which the federal government promoted growth and consolidation during the 1960s. As they observed at the time:

> *The health system should be re-created as a democratic enterprise, in which patients are participants (not customers or objects) and the health workers, from physicians to aides, are all colleagues in a common undertaking.* [6]

That warning has come to pass since then, with rapid growth of health care corporations, increased privatization, corporatized markets, shift to for-profit health care as a commodity, and weakening of the doctor-patient relationship. As we saw in the first chapter (Figures 1.2 and 1.3), for-profit ownership became dominant across the medical-industrial complex, together with soaring growth in numbers of administrators compared to physicians.

In the course of all of these changes, health care became less of a public good as it morphed into a profiteering machine increasingly controlled by Wall Street traders and investors. Private equity drove investment based on profits without regard to quality of care, which was compromised, as was documented in the last chapter (Table 3.1).

The extent of these changes is reflected in Table 4.1, showing how the mission and values of publicizers (such as policy-oriented health planning persons in government) differ from privatizers (such as a CEO of a market-oriented HMO). [7]

Claire Fagin, dean emerita of the School of Nursing at the University of Pennsylvania, had this to say about these momentous changes in health care:

> *Markets are amoral in general, that is sentimentally neutral, but in health care this general amorality has the potential to become immoral.*
>
> *The buyers, industry, and government want to reduce costs. The sellers, the managed care organizations, must reduce costs to remain competitive and provide profits to shareholders. Caregivers become implicit and explicit rationers of care who often benefit directly from rationing, a factor that is unique in the American system and exists nowhere else in the industrialized world.* [8]

TABLE 4.1

A COMPARISON OF PUBLICIZER AND PRIVATIZER VIEWS

Issue	Publicizer View	Privatizer View
Problem with current system	Public interests ill-served: Too many uninsured Costs too high Too much private profiteering	Market distorted by: Tax policy Risk selection in small-group, individual markets Excessive regulation
Highest values	Equity, predictability, security, control	Efficiency/effectiveness, flexibility, speed, change
Nature of beneficiary	Vulnerable, needs to be protected	Customer, needs to be satisfied
Price competition in health care	Cannot work	Is the only way
Favorite federal health program	Medicare	FEHBP
Successful health plan	Meets one goal: High-quality service at reasonable cost	Meets two goals: Attracts capital Attracts customers
Management focus	Cost and consistency Constituencies Motives and effort	Price and value Buyers and competitors Results
Managed care abuses	Make them illegal	Market will weed out
Providers and insurers	Suppliers or thieves (maybe both)	Partners or competitors (maybe both)
Who assures integrity of health plans?	Inspector general and audit army	Buyers/consumers with choices
Profit	Tolerable only at low level	Essential fuel; earn or die
Accounting statement	Every line	Bottom line
Conflict of interest	Should be a disqualifying condition	Get it on the table; take it into account
Insurance rating	Community rating; spread the risks	Large group experience; reward smart buyers
Insurance benefits	National standard benefit package, in splendid detail	Let markets decide; standardize only within accounts
Best allocator of resources	Public body backed by technically competent planning agency	The "invisible hand"
Approach to health care reform	Comprehensive; balance conflicting interests	Incremental; improve market dynamics

Note: FEHBP is Federal Employees Health Benefits Program.

Source: Reprinted with permission from Cain HP. *Privatizing Medicare: A battle of values. Health Affairs* (Millwood). 1997;16(2):185

As a result of this fundamental transformation in a corporatized market in U. S. health care, we have seen these uninterrupted detrimental changes that have been resistant to reversal:

- prices to what the traffic will bear;
- uncontained costs;
- decreased choice and access to care;
- compromised quality of care, with worse outcomes;
- rampant profiteering and fraud; and
- weak oversight by government with little accountability.

In their 2000 publication *Health and Health Care 2010: The Forecast, The Challenges,* the Institute of the Future predicted stormy weather for 2010 (Figure 4.1), all of which has come to pass. [9] Although the ACA of 2010 helped to improve access to care around the edges, it has been completely unsuccessful in containing health care costs or reversing the above fundamental transformative system changes.

I. Corruption of Honored Health Professions by the Invisible Hand of a Non-Caring Corporatized Marketplace

The largely deregulated market over the last 40 years has been driven by profits over quality and service, with consolidation of the major players leading to oligopoly and often tacit rate setting by large corporate interests. Here we consider four of these players.

1. Private health insurers

Long past their early history with a mission of service through a social insurance model, the Blues and other private health insurers have largely abandoned that mission for the business "ethic" of maximizing profits for themselves and their shareholders on Wall Street. After the entry of large for-profit private insurers into the health care market during the 1970s and 1980s, Blue Cross and Blue Shield were forced to go for-profit in 1994 in order to better compete. [10]

FIGURE 4.1

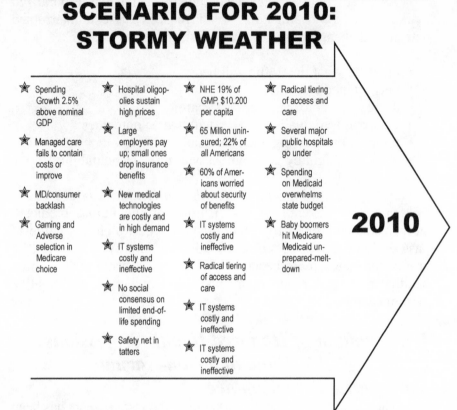

SCENARIO FOR 2010: STORMY WEATHER

☆ Spending Growth 2.5% above nominal GDP

☆ Managed care fails to contain costs or improve

☆ MD/consumer backlash

☆ Gaming and Adverse selection in Medicare choice

☆ Hospital oligop-olies sustain high prices

☆ Large employers pay up; small ones drop insurance benefits

☆ New medical technologies are costly and in high demand

☆ IT systems costly and ineffective

☆ No social consensus on limited end-of-life spending

☆ Safety net in tatters

☆ NHE 19% of GMP, $10.200 per capita

☆ 65 Million unin-sured; 22% of all Americans

☆ 60% of Amer-icans worried about security of benefits

☆ IT systems costly and ineffective

☆ Radical tiering of access and care

☆ IT systems costly and ineffective

☆ IT systems costly and ineffective

☆ Radical tiering of access and care

☆ Several major public hospitals go under

☆ Spending on Medicaid overwhelms state budget

☆ Baby boomers hit Medicare Medicaid un-prepared-melt-down

2010

Source: *Health and Health Care 2010: The Forecast, the Challenge, The Institute for the Future*, San Francisco, CA. *Jossey-Bass*, 2003

Today, private insurers have many ways to raise higher revenues on the backs of enrollees, including deceptive marketing, avoiding sicker enrollees, denial of services, churning of networks, and exiting unprofitable markets. To show how successful these practices are in terms of revenues, the seven largest publicly traded health insurers grew their profits by a combined 66 percent from 2018 to 2019. Most of this profiteering was driven by deals with other health-related businesses, such as pharmacies and pharmacy benefit managers (PBMs). After Cigna acquired the PBM Express Scripts, its revenue surged by 216 percent within the following year. Beyond mergers and acquisitions, the big health insurers also gain by continuing membership growth in Medicare Advantage and Medicaid. [11]

2. Privatized public programs, with loss of social contract

Medicare Advantage and Medicaid have been a bonanza for private insurers, now accounting for more than one-half of their net revenue, as we saw in Figure 1.1 (page 10). Insurers have successfully lobbied Congress over the years for higher payments, and have also fraudulently increased their payments by up-coding diagnoses—by exaggerating how sick their enrollees are and/or claiming payment for conditions for which treatment was not given. [12] Insurers have been partnering with third-party vendors to perform medical chart reviews to find thousands of extra diagnostic codes that can be claimed for overpayments. [13] Figure 4.2 shows how these large overpayments increased between 2008 and 2016, with a surge of up-coding after passage of the ACA in 2010. [14]

FIGURE 4.2

MEDICARE OVERPAYS PRIVATE PLANS

Total Overpayments 2008-2016: $173.7 billion

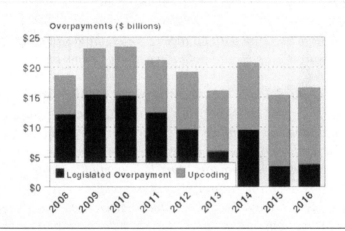

Source: PNHP Report 10/20/12 - based on data from MedPAC, *Comonwealth Fund*, Trivedi et al.

Although both Medicare and Medicaid were established as a social contract with their enrollees, both have strayed from this purpose the more they have become privatized. These two typical patient experiences illustrate how far that betrayal has gone today:

When Ed Stein turned 65, he was active and healthy. He chose a Medicare Advantage plan instead of traditional Medicare, attracted by the extra benefits and unaware of how difficult it would be later to switch over to public Medicare. After being diagnosed with an aggressive bladder cancer at 72, he had to undergo chemotherapy and a complex surgical procedure. That was when he learned that the surgeon he wanted to see was out of network, and when he found that it was impossible then to switch back to Medicare in order to have full choice of physician and hospital. [Many people at 65 sign up for supplemental coverage through Medigap, which cannot reject you in the first 6 months, but can thereafter for pre-existing conditions.] Ed had to scramble to find where to go and whom to see, including a last-minute switch to another Medicare Advantage plan with his preferred surgeon in network. His search ended up with treatment at four different hospitals. As his wife said after this ordeal: "When you're in the middle of a health crisis, the last thing you need is to be negotiating with health providers and insurance. We spent as many hours talking with all these people about squaring away our insurance as we did actually getting treatment." [15]

Rasha Salama has taken her two children to Dr. Inas Wassef, a pediatrician who speaks her native language, Arabic, and has an office just a few blocks from her home in a blue-collar community across the bay from New York City. As she says of her doctor, "She knows my kids, answers the phone, is open on Saturdays and is everything for me." But enter giant UnitedHealthcare and that care ended abruptly. It is dropping hundreds of doctors in its central and northern New Jersey Medicaid physician network, forcing thousands of patients to leave their longtime physicians. This kind of move has become common as insurers narrow their networks of physicians to others with practice patterns easier to control. [16]

Dr. Bernard Lown, developer of the cardiac defibrillator and co-recipient of the Nobel Peace Prize in 1985 on behalf of International Physicians for the Prevention of Nuclear War, said this in 1998 as the medical-industrial complex was enveloping medicine and health care:

The United States subscribes to a business model that characterizes insurers as commercial entities. Like all businesses, their goal is to make money ... Under the business model, casual inhumanity is built in and the common good ignored. Excluding the poor, the aged, the disabled and the ill is sound policy since it maximizes profit. Under the social model, denying coverage to any member of society would refute the fundamental purpose of health insurance. [17]

3. Consolidation of larger hospital systems and physician practices

This is another major trend disrupting relationships among hospitals, physicians, and patients. According to Avalere Health and the Physicians Advisory Institute, hospitals acquired some 8,000 medical practices, and 14,000 physicians left private practice to work in hospitals between 2016 and 2018. Amidst this turmoil, more independent physician practices are now looking to private equity to grow and compete in this rapidly changing marketplace. As expected, private equity firms are especially interested in such well-reimbursed specialties as dermatology, orthopedic surgery and gastroenterology. As one example, only 6,000 of the 14,500 gastroenterologists in the country are still in private practice.[18] Further disarray of medical practice is happening as the largest health insurers buy up physician practices and steer patients to clinics that they own. [19]

II. Can Conservatives Hold to Their Principles and still Support Universal Health Care?

Conservatives in most other advanced countries around the world have long supported universal access to necessary health care on the basis of these four conservative moral principles: *anti-free riding, personal integrity, equal opportunity*, and *just sharing.* Donald Light, Ph.D, as a Fellow at the University of Pennsylvania's Center for Bioethics and author of *Benchmarks for Fairness for Health Care Reform*, suggested these ten guidelines in 2002 for conservatives to hold to these principles:

"1. Everyone is covered, and everyone contributes in proportion to his or her income.
2. Decisions about all matters are open and publicly debated. Accountability for costs, quality, and value of providers, suppliers, and administrators is public.
3. Contributions do not discriminate by type of illness or ability to pay.
4. Coverage does not discriminate by type of illness or ability to pay.
5. Coverage responds first to medical need and suffering.
6. Nonfinancial barriers by class, language, education, and geography are to be minimized.
7. Providers are paid fairly and equitably, taking into account their local circumstances.
8. Clinical waste is minimized through public health, self-care, prevention, strong primary care, and identification of unnecessary procedures.
9. Financial waste is minimized through simplified administrative arrangements and strong bargaining for good value.
10. Choice is maximized in a common playing field where 90-95 percent of payments go toward necessary and efficient health services and only 5-10 percent to administration." [20]

Conclusion:

A fundamental transformation of medicine and health care has occurred over the last 60 years from an honored profession and related health care fields committed to service to patients and communities—to what it has become—taken over in the drive to profits for corporations and investors. Health care has become just another commodity in a largely for-profit health care marketplace where there is hardly time or priority left for personhood or the physician-patient relationship.

Profiteering and invisible fraud have become the new normal in U. S. health care. Shannon Brownlee and Dr. Vikas Saini of the Lown Institute noted in 2017 how such practices as industry payouts to providers, unnecessary hospital admissions to meet quotas, and manipulating data for greater reimbursements had become the new normal in a corrupt system. As they said at the time,

Our health care system is no longer about relieving the suffering of patients or the intrinsic value of maintaining the health of our population. It's about making money. [21]

That observation is especially pertinent as we move into Part II, where we will examine the many ways that patients lose every day in our profit-driven system that so often fails to meet their needs.

References:

1. Relman, AS. Medical professionalism in a commercialized health care market. *JAMA* 298 (22): 2669, 2007.
2. Johnston, DC. *The Big Print: How Big Companies Use "Plain English" to Rob You Blind*. New York. *Penguin Group*, 2013: p. 26.
3. Falk, IS. Some lessons from the fifty years since the COMC Final Report, 1932. *J Public Health Policy* 4 (2): 139, 1983.
4. Starr, P. *The Social Transformation of American Medicine: The Rise of a Sovereign Profession and the Making of a Vast Industry*. New York. *Basic Books*, 1982, p. 295.
5. McNerney, W. C Rufus Rorem award lecture. Big question for the Blues: Where to go from here? *Inquiry*. (Summer): 33: 110-117, 1996.
6. Ehrenreich, B and J. The Medical Industrial Complex. Review of book by Ginsberg, E (with Ostow, M) *Men, Money and Medicine. The New York Review of Books*. New York. Columbia, 1970.
7. Cain, HP. Privatizing Medicare: A battle of values. *Health Affairs (Millwood)* 16 (2): 181-186, 1997.
8. Fagin, CM. Two American taboos: Criticizing the market and supporting universal health care. *Nursing Leadership Forum*. Winter 4 (2): 50, 1999.
9. Institute for the Future. *Health and Health Care 2010: The Forecast, the Challenges*. San Francisco, CA. *Jossey-Bass*, 2000.
10. Reich, RB. *The Common Good*. New York. *Alfred A. Knopf*, 2018, p. 80.
11. Livingston, S. Insurers reaped big financial gains from mergers in 2019. *Modern Healthcare*, February 24, 2020.
12. Livingston, S. Insurers profit from Medicare Advantage's incentive to add coding that boosts reimbursement. *Modern Healthcare*, September 4, 2018.
13. Schulte, F, Weber, L. Medicare Advantage overbills taxpayers by billions a year as feds struggle to stop it. *Kaiser Health News*, July 16, 2019.
14. Geruso, M, Layton, T. Up-coding inflates Medicare costs in excess of $2 billion annually. *UT News*, University of Texas at Austin, June 18, 2015.
15. Miller, M. Medicare's private option is gaining popularity, and critics. *New York Times*, February 21, 2020.
16. Galewitz, P. Needy patients 'caught in the middle' as insurance titan drops doctors. *Kaiser Health News*, February 25, 2020.

17. Lown, B. Physicians need to fight the business model of medicine. *Hippocrates* 12 (5): 25-28, 1998.
18. Suthrum, P. Physician practice consolidation: It's only just begun. STAT, February 27, 2020.
19. Mathews, AW. Physicians, hospitals meet their new competitor: insurer-owned clinics. *Wall Street Journal*, February 23, 2020.
20. Light, DW. A conservative call for universal access to health care. *Penn Bioeth J* 9 (4): 4-6, 2002.
21. Saini, V, Brownlee, S. As quoted by Garber, J. Why corruption is the new normal in health care (and what we can do about it. *The Lown Institute*, June 1, 2017.

PART II

ADVERSE IMPACTS OF THESE HISTORICAL CHANGES ON PATIENTS AND THE U. S. POPULATION

The notion of price control is anathema to health care companies. It threatens their basic business model, in which the government grants them approvals and patents, pays whatever they ask, and works hand in hand with them as they deliver the worst health outcomes at the highest costs in the rich world.

The American health care industry is not good at promoting health but it excels at taking money from all of us for its benefit. It is an engine of inequality.

—Anne Case, Ph.D. and Angus Deaton, Ph.D, Professors emeritus of Economics and Public Affairs, Princeton University, and coauthors of *Deaths of Despair and the Future of Capitalism.* [1]

(1) Case, A, Deaton, A. America can afford a world-class health system. Why don't we have one? *New York Times, April 14, 2020.*

Chapter 5

DECREASED ACCESS TO UNAFFORDABLE CARE

As we have already seen, most of the U. S. health care system is profit-driven, with unrestrained prices and costs of health care services. It is time now to question what impacts these have had on access to care. The goals of this chapter are: (1) to assess the magnitude of increasing health care costs and prices; (2) to describe some of the many ways whereby patients find health care costs unaffordable; and (3) to briefly discuss the implications of how we ration care based on ability to pay.

I. Soaring Health Care Prices and Costs: How Bad Are They?

The costs of health insurance and health care have been rising for many years at rates far above the inflation rate or cost of living, to the point that they now are an unsustainable level that consumes almost one-half of the average household income for a family of four. Despite the passage of the ACA ten years ago, these prices and costs have not been reined in as the free-wheeling health care marketplace barrels along, rewarding corporate stakeholders and Wall Street investors at the expense of patients, families and taxpayers.

The Milliman Medical Index (MMI) is one of the best markers for tracking the continuing explosion of health care costs for individuals and families. Its 2019 report found that the average individual American now spends $6,348 a year for health care, while the average hypothetical family of four with an employer-sponsored PPO plan pays $28,386 a year, almost one-half of the median U. S. household income. That includes premiums, cost-sharing, and forgone wage increases (for the employer contribution). Figure 5.1 shows how the MMI has grown from 2001 to 2019 in this country. [1]

FIGURE 5.1

MILLIMAN MEDICAL INDEX, 2001-2019

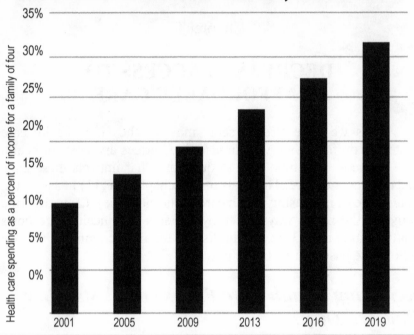

Source: *Milliman Research Report*, July 25, 2019

Health care costs and prices are being driven by these inter-related pressures—high administrative overhead, waste, lack of price controls, profiteering, corruption and fraud that remain beyond control across the medical-industrial complex. Our market-driven system has consolidated to the point that a small number of corporate stakeholders with large market shares can charge what the traffic will bear. Figure 5.2 shows how the CPI for medical costs has been accelerating compared to the consumer-price index over the last 25 years. [2]

At this same time, the costs of all kinds of health insurance are rising rapidly, even as they cover less. Figure 5.3 shows the annual growth of spending for private insurance, Medicare and Medicaid from 2012 to 2018. The net cost of private insurance jumped by more than 15 percent in 2018, the biggest increase since 2003. [3]

Each of these kinds of insurance will cost more for less coverage through increased cost-sharing and more out-of-pocket (OOP) costs. The Commonwealth Fund has found that almost 24 million Americans with employer-sponsored coverage have high

FIGURE 5.2

INCREASING BURDEN OF HEALTH CARE COSTS, 1980 - PRESENT

As the cost of medical care rises, states' promises to provide health care to their employees in retirement are growing increasingly burdensome.

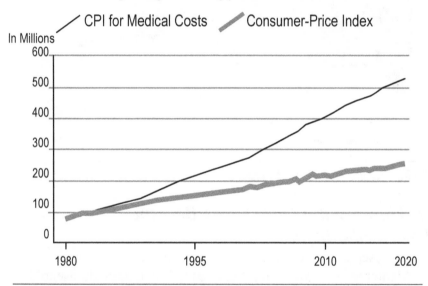

Source: Federal Reserve Bank of St. Louis

premium contributions or high OOP costs relative to income, or both. [4] Employer-based insurance, as the largest source of health insurance, gives considerably less financial protection than those with coverage on an ACA market plan. [5] According to a recent report from the Health Care Cost Institute, the increasing costs of commercial insurance are being driven by higher prices of health care services, as illustrated by these two examples:

- the average OOP price for an emergency room visit went up from $368 in 2014 to $503 in 2018.
- the average price of infusion drugs administered in physicians' clinics soared 73 percent from 2014 to 2018. [6]

FIGURE 5.3

ANNUAL GROWTH OF SPENDING FOR PRIVATE INSURANCE, MEDICARE AND MEDICAID, 2012-2018

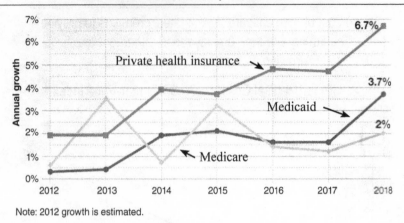

Note: 2012 growth is estimated.

Source: *Health Affairs*, 39, No 1, 2020

II. How Health Care Costs Become Unaffordable for Patients and Families

According to a recent report from the Centers for Medicare and Medicaid Services (CMS), U.S. household spending on health care topped $1 trillion for the first time in 2018. [7] Another recent study found that patients' OOP costs for inpatient hospital services increased on average by 14 percent between 2017 and 2018. [8]

It is instructive to see how these numbers relate to what patients and their families experience as they try to deal with this unsustainable problem, now the number one domestic issue in the current debates in the 2020 election cycle. For them, the numbers are far from abstract, but serious day-to-day challenges. These are some of their biggest challenges, even when insured, as patients try to navigate a changing landscape filled with financial barriers to care.

1. Increased cost-sharing and OOP costs

Figure 5.4 shows how premiums and deductibles have climbed over the last ten years, much above workers' wages. The average deductible for a single worker with employer-based insurance rose from just $379 in 2006 to $1,350 in 2018. The average total cost for an employer-based family plan reached $20,576 in 2019, with employees paying about one-third of that cost. [9] Many people have worse plans with much higher deductibles that force them to forego or delay care.

FIGURE 5.4

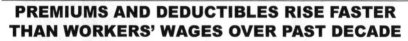

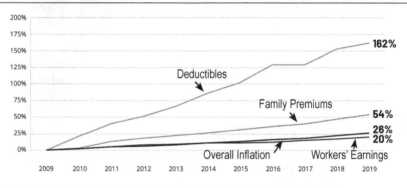

Source: Kaiser Family Foundation, and Bureau of Labor Statistics

Four in ten people with job-based health insurance report that they don't have enough savings to cover the deductible, while one in six have to take an extra job, cut back on food, or move in with friends or family. [10] Figure 5.5 shows how high deductibles cut access to care across the board. As Dr. Veena Shankaran of the Hutchinson Cancer Research Center in Seattle notes:

High-deductible plans are really the epitome of the access to care problem. People don't have the liquid cash to meet the deductible, so you see delays in care or even avoiding treatment altogether. [11]

FIGURE 5.5

HIGH DEDUCTIBLES CUT
ALL KINDS OF CARE

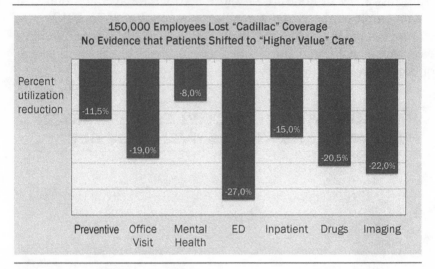

150,000 Employees Lost "Cadillac" Coverage
No Evidence that Patients Shifted to "Higher Value" Care

Percent utilization reduction: -11,5% (Preventive), -19,0% (Office Visit), -8,0% (Mental Health), -27,0% (ED), -15,0% (Inpatient), -20,5% (Drugs), -22,0% (Imaging)

Source: Brot-Goldberg et al, 6/2015

Here are two typical patients' stories that illustrate this problem, even for those with solid middle annual incomes.

Andrew Holko, a 45-year-old father of two is facing $5,000 in outstanding medical bills because of diabetes medications, cortisone injections for his wife's needs for pelvic pain, a recent trip to the emergency room for his 9-year-old daughter and other services. Although his household income from his information technology job is above $80,000, close to the median for a family of four, he has little extra to cover a $4,000 annual deductible and still pay for a mortgage, two growing children, and student loans. As he says: "We shop at discount grocery stores. My wife is couponing. We are putting every single bill we can on the credit card. Even a family meal at McDonald's seems like a luxury. We're drowning."

Tomas Krusliak, a 27-year-old chef in western Virginia, took on two extra jobs, working some days from 5 a.m. to 11 p.m., to pay medical bills after his wife had a miscarriage as the couple tried to have their first baby. They had a $5,000 deductible. Originally from Slovakia, he said this about his experience here: "I was used to having insurance where I could go to the doctor and get the treatment I needed. It was definitely a shock when I got to the U. S. and learned that even when you are working and getting insurance, you have to spend even more money to get treatment. [12]

2. Can't shop for value of care

It is very difficult, often impossible, to get estimated costs of a medical service that is being planned, especially since costs and prices are not transparent and providers themselves usually don't know. These estimates are frequently far from the final bill, which is always on the high side. Here is one typical couple's experience with now widespread surprise medical bills.

Rebecca Grimm, 29, and her husband Mark tried to shop for the best price for a surgical procedure when she had a miscarriage in 2018. With a high deductible plan, she first tried to clear the tissue with a $10 pill. When that failed, she checked the cost of a surgical procedure at several local medical centers. The estimates were all about $900, she had the 20-minute procedure done a few miles from their home, but later she received a bill for $5,948. [13]

3. Inadequacy and instability of health insurance

Employer-based insurance

These plans cost more all the time for employers and employees, including foregone wage increases. Some 66 million people left their jobs in 2018, then had to find other work, with or without health benefits, and had no insurance while job hunting. The average person these days has 12 jobs before age 50. [14] Low income families (below twice the federal poverty level) with job-based insurance are spending 14 percent of their income on premiums and OOP costs, much more than the 8.4 percent being paid by their counterparts with ACA market coverage. [15]

This patient's story is unfortunately very common:

> *Jessie McCormick, 27, with a heart condition and working full-time at a nonprofit in Washington, calculated that her OOP costs would be at least $1,200 a month to cover her medical expenses, double the money left over after paying her rent and utilities. In order to deal with these costs, she left her job in order to qualify for Medicaid that would cover her medical expenses.* [16]

Medicare

One might think that traditional Medicare would cover most of the costs of essential care, but that is far from true. While it does cover 80 percent of hospital and physicians' services for hospitalizations, there are many areas for which it does not provide coverage, such as vision, hearing, dental, and drug coverage. An analysis by the Kaiser Family Foundation recently found that the average person with traditional Medicare spent $5,460 in OOP payments for health care in 2016.

Figure 5.6 shows that Medicare households with members 85 and older spent 40% of their budgets on health-related expenses in 2016. [17]

FIGURE 5.6

PROPORTION OF SPENDING ON HEALTH-RELATED EXPENSES FOR MEDICARE HOUSEHOLDS WITH MEMBERS AGED 85 AND OLDER, 2016

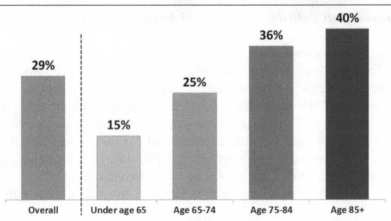

Source: Kaiser Family Foundation, and the Bureau of Labor Statistics, 2016

Medicare Advantage

In order to gain broader coverage, many seniors purchase supplemental Medigap plans through private insurers or are attracted to privatized Medicare Advantage. But this "coverage" is often absent, as this patient found out the hard way.

> *Tom Mills, 71, a retired environmental geologist in San Diego with a Medicare Advantage plan, suffered a mild stroke with no lasting effects after a mitral valve repair. He soon learned that OOP costs for future care would soar now that he had a pre-existing condition. He considered shifting back to traditional Medicare plus supplemental Medigap, but was advised by an insurance broker that no supplemental plan would take him due to this new pre-existing condition, despite being in training for his 57th half marathon!* [18]

Though initially attracting enrollees with attractive premiums, Medicare Advantage dis-enrolls them at the drop of a hat when they get sick. For individuals wanting to return to traditional Medicare and a prescription drug plan, they would still need a supplemental Medigap plan to cover the 20 percent copays and deductibles. But once past the first 12 months after reaching age 65, Medigap policies are not required to provide coverage, and if they do, it would be with prohibitive premiums if one had pre-existing conditions. [19]

Medicaid

Although Medicaid serves as an important safety net program in many states, eligibility varies greatly from one state to another. The overall thrust of the Trump administration is to reduce and weaken the ACA's Medicaid expansion and cut back on eligibility and enrollment, especially through state waivers. These waivers can allow states to impose premiums and other kinds of cost sharing, work requirements. [20] Alabama is an extremely restrictive state where those with annual incomes more than 18 percent of the federal poverty level are not eligible for Medicaid. [21] Moreover, there is a high level of churning of coverage in many states as enrollees change circumstances and incomes.

ACA market plans

Despite the ACA's partial reduction in the numbers of uninsured over the last ten years, mostly through Medicaid expansion, there are still 87 million Americans who are underinsured. [22] The

Commonwealth Fund defines underinsurance as spending more than 10 % of annual income on health care, more than 5% of income if below 200 % of the federal poverty level, or deductibles equal to or exceeding 5% of income.

Short-term plans

These plans, correctly labeled as "junk insurance," get around the ACA's requirements in providing very limited coverage at exorbitant costs for up to a year. Golden Rule Insurance is aptly named for bringing big profits to its owner, UnitedHealth Group. [23]

Insurer won't cover drug prescribed by physician

Although most health insurers claim to include prescription drug coverage, a recent national poll found that these insurers deny covering prescriptions for more than one-third of adults across all income groups. In almost one-half of these denials, the prescriptions were never filled. [24]

Long-term care insurance

As the costs and claims for long-term care have spiraled upward, the number of insurers offering coverage has dropped precipitously. Among the few remaining insurers, benefits are restricted and premiums are unaffordable for many seniors and people with disabilities. Medicare provides little coverage for long-term care, while Medicaid covers more of its costs, but only after patients have spent down to poverty level.

4. Narrowed networks

The growing number of mergers and consolidation, especially among hospital systems that also include purchase of medical practices, typically leads to narrowed networks that disrupt continuity of care and previous coverage of hospital and physician services. As a result, prices go up and costs become unaffordable for many patients receiving care by out-of-network providers. This has been a common cause of staggering surprise medical bills. A recent study by researchers at Yale University put real numbers to this problem—hospital-based specialists, especially anesthesiologists, assistant surgeons, radiologists and pathologists, boost spending by $40 billion annually. Out-of-network assistant surgeons were the biggest culprit, charging more than 25 times average Medicare rates! [25] Networks are constantly changing as insurers renegotiate arrangements with hospitals and physicians, leaving insured patients often unaware of what is and isn't covered and at risk for surprise medical bills. [26]

III. Rationing by Ability to Pay

The ACA didn't help as much as its celebrants claim—no cost containment, still 30 million uninsured, 87 million underinsured, and all the problems getting care even if insured, as described previously. Despite a modest improvement in access to care after the ACA of 2010, a recent study of unmet needs for U. S. adults ages 18 to 64 years between 1998 and 2018 drew these conclusions:

- "most measures of unmet need for physician services have shown no improvement, and financial access to physician services has decreased;
- the rise of narrow networks, high-deductible plans, and higher co-pays has contributed to the growth of unmet medical needs in the U. S. since the 1990s; and
- our findings call into question the value of private insurance today, when it fails to ensure that health care is affordable when needed." [27]

In fact, a 2020 report from the American Hospital Association found that hospital outpatient visits just dropped for the first time in 35 years. [28]

With the most expensive health care system in the world, the U. S. severely rations care by ability to pay—unfair, unjust, and against public and societal interests. In their 2020 book, *Deaths of Despair and the Future of Capitalism*, Drs. Anne Case and Angus Deaton, Professors emeritus of Economics and Public Affairs at Princeton University, argue that U. S. households pay an extra $8,000 a year compared with what Swiss families pay in the second most expensive system in the world—in effect, amounting to a "poll tax" regardless of ability to pay. [29]

The stakes of increasing unaffordability of health care in this country could not be higher—probably higher than many people realize. People are dying from this growing problem. A recent national study by Gallup and West Health, a non-profit organization, found that 34 million adults know someone who has died after not getting necessary care because of its unaffordability. It also found that 58 million adults reported their inability to pay for needed medicine or drugs prescribed by their physicians. [30]

The U. S. is now challenged by the COVID-19 pandemic, with the largest number of cases and deaths in any country around the world. We can expect that health care costs will become even less affordable, with more delayed and foregone care than ever. Amidst a deepening recession or even depression, Medicaid programs will experience increased enrollment as the ranks of the unemployed grow, already passing 36 million at this writing. [31]

We need a strong safety net for Americans who cannot afford care, and it is in tatters as the health care gravy train rolls on in our corporatized system. The late Dr. Uwe Reinhardt, Ph.D., well-known Professor of Political Economy, Economics and Public Affairs at Princeton University and author of the 2019 book, *Priced Out: The Economic and Ethical Costs of American Health Care*, had this to say on the subject:

> *Our financing of health care is really a moral morass. It is a moral morass in the sense that it signals to the doctors and hospitals that human beings have different values depending on their income status. To give you a specific example, in New Jersey, the Medicaid program pays a pediatrician $30 to see a poor child on Medicaid. But the same legislators, through their commercial insurance, pay the same pediatrician $100 to $120 to see their child . . . How do physicians react to it? If you phone around practices in Princeton, Plainsboro, Hamilton, as I did for 15 practices—none of them would see Medicaid kids.*
>
> *So here you have a country that often relies on these kids to fight their wars, and yet treats them as if they were lower-value human beings through the payment system. I think that is unique. No other country would make a differentiation like that. So that's a disgrace.* [32]

Conclusion:

We will return in Chapter 8 to describe in more detail the extent of profiteering, waste, corruption and fraud within our system, followed in Chapter 9 by the harms caused to patients, health professionals, and taxpayers as a result of these excesses. For now, however, we turn to the next chapter to consider what all this means to the quality of health care that Americans receive, or don't receive.

References:

1. Milliman. Healthcare costs reach $6,348 for the average American, $28,386 for hypothetical family of four. *Milliman Research Report*, July 25, 2019.
2. Gillers, H. Retiree health benefits cut. *Wall Street Journal*, May 2, 2019.
3. Meyer, H. Growth in medical prices inched healthcare spending higher in 2018. *Modern Healthcare*, December 9, 2019.
4. Hayes, SL, Collins, SR, Radley, DC. How much U. S. households with employer-insurance spend on premiums and out-of-pocket costs: A state-by-state look. *The Commonwealth Fund*, May 23, 2019.
5. Altman, D. For low-income people, employer health coverage is worse than ACA. *Axios*, April 15, 2019.
6. Herman, B. Health care prices still rising faster than use of services. *Axios*, February 14, 2020.
7. Luhby, T. U. S. household spending on health care tops $1 trillion in 2028 for first time. *CNN Politics*, December 5, 2019.
8. Bannow, T. Report: Patients' out-of-pocket costs for inpatient services increased by 14 % on average between 2017 and 2018. *Modern Healthcare*, June 25, 2019.
9. Mathews, AW. Cost of employer health plans jumps. *Wall Street Journal*, September 26, 2019.
10. Levey, NN. Health insurance deductibles soar, leaving Americans with unaffordable bills. *Los Angeles Times,* May 2, 2019.
11. Shankaran, V. As quoted by Stallings, E. High-deductible health policies linked to delayed diagnosis and treatment. *NPR*, April 18, 2019.
12. Ibid # 11.
13. Levey, NN. Trying to shop for medical care? Lots of luck with that. *Los Angeles Times*, October 1, 2019.
14. Bruenig, M. People lose their employer-sponsored insurance constantly. *People's Policy Project*, April 4, 2019.
15. Altman, D. For low-income people, employer health coverage is worse than ACA. *Axios*, April 15, 2019.
16. Abelson, R. Employer health insurance is increasingly unaffordable, study finds. *New York Times*, September 25, 2019.
17. Medicare beneficiaries spent an average of $5,460 out of pocket for health care in 2016, with some groups spending substantially more. *Kaiser Family Foundation*, November 4, 2019.
18. Clark, C. Medicare Advantage enrollees discover dirty little secret: Getting out is a lot harder than getting in. *MedPage Today*, December 3, 2019.
19. Ibid # 18.
20. Bernstein, J. Katch, H. Trump administration's under-the-radar attack on Medicaid is gaining speed. *The Washington Post*, March 6, 2018.

21. Cunningham, PW. Here are three big ways the Trump administration could put its mark on Medicaid. *The Washington Post*, May 16, 2018.

22. Collins, SR, Bhupal, HK, Doty, MM. Health insurance coverage eight years after the ACA. *The Commonwealth Fund*, February 7, 2019.

23. Hiltzik, M. Why the short-term health plans are cheap: They shortchange you on care. *Los Angeles Times*, August 12, 2019.

24. Neighmond, P. When insurance won't cover drugs, Americans make 'tough choices' about their health. *NPR*, January 27, 2020.

25. Livingston, S. Out of network billing by hospital-based specialists boosts spending by $40 billion. *Modern Healthcare*, December 16, 2019.

26. Minemyer, P. BlueCross Blue Shield Association shifting support to narrower network plans. *FierceHealthcare*, November 13, 2019.

27. Hawks, L, Himmelstein, DU, Woolhandler, S et al. Trends in unmet need for physician and preventive services in the United States, 1998-2017. *JAMA Internal Medicine,* January 27, 2020.

28. Bannow, T. As competition heats up, hospital outpatient visits see first dip in 35 years. *Modern Healthcare*, January 13, 2020.

29. Long, H. Health-care costs are like an $8,000 'tax' on every family, economists say. *The Washington Post,* January 8, 2020: A20.

30. Curtin, A. New study shows staggering consequences of for-profit healthcare system and Americans' inability to pay for it. *Nation of Change*, November 16, 2019.

31. Cox, C, Rudowitz, R, Neuman, T et all. How health costs may change with COVID-19. *Peterson-KFF Health System Tracker*, April 15, 2020.

32. Reinhardt, UE. *Priced Out: The Economic and Ethical Costs of American Health Care*. Princeton, NJ. *Princeton University Press*, 2019, pp. 161-162.

Chapter 6

WORSE QUALITY OF CARE

As we saw in the last chapter, the U. S. severely rations care based on ability to pay. If people can't afford its high prices, they often delay or forego care altogether. Restricted access leads to worse quality of care and outcomes for many millions of Americans, but there is another problem on the other side of the equation—overutilization, with about one-third of health care services unnecessary, inappropriate, and sometimes harmful. [1,2]

In his 2019 book, *The Great Reversal: How America Gave Up on Free Markets*, Thomas Philippon, Professor of Finance at the Stern School of Business at New York University, gets our attention with this overview of the U. S. health care system after study of health care elsewhere in the world:

> *The gap between what we could do and what we actually do is much greater than the rate of technological change over at least several decades. The U. S. has the best hospitals and the best technologies, yet it has mediocre health outcomes. An inefficient, oligopolistic and sometimes corrupt health care system is not the only reason, but it is a major contributor. . . The U. S. is experiencing the first peacetime decline of life expectancy of any democratic nation since the Industrial Revolution.* [3]

In order to better understand what is going on in this country with quality of health care, this chapter has three goals: (1) to describe ways by which our profit-driven system compromises quality of care; (2) to see how our system compares with international and U. S. state measures of health care; and (3) to briefly consider what can be done to improve our system's quality of care.

I. Ways in which our profit-driven system compromises quality of care

First, let's get some overall numbers as to what has been happening in recent years. Our 30 million uninsured Americans, together with 87 million underinsured, clearly have difficulty in accessing care when needed. A 2019 Gallup poll found that one-third of Americans reported that their family could not afford care in the past year, with one in four deferring care for a serious condition.[4] Figure 6.1 shows the types of care that are delayed or forgone because of unaffordable costs. Figure 6.2 that many of the uninsured who lack a usual source of care are more likely to forego preventive care.

FIGURE 6.1

PERCENT OF ADULTS WHO REPORT DELAYING AND/OR GOING WITHOUT MEDICAL CARE DUE TO COSTS, BY TYPE OF CARE, 2016

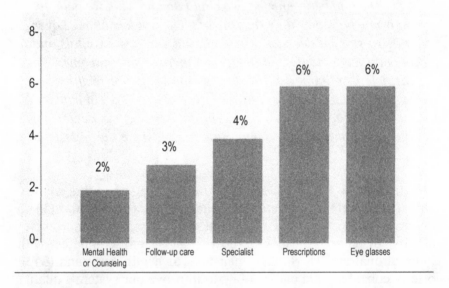

Source: Kaiser Family Foundation analysis of National Health Interview Survey. Peterson-Kaiser Health System Tracker.

FIGURE 6.2

UNINSURED ADULTS WHO LACK A USUAL SOURCE OF CARE ARE ALSO MORE LIKELY TO FORGO PREVENTIVE CARE

Percent of adults who did not report a usual source of care, who reported going without preventive care, 2016

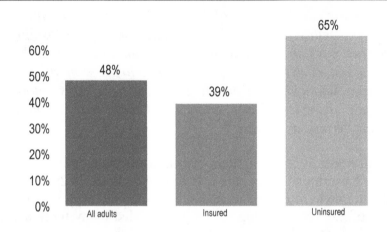

Source: Kaiser Family Foundation analysis of National Health Interview Survey. Peterson-Kaiser Health System Tracker.

The Trump administration has been expanding the numbers of underinsured by its promotion of short-term plans that have attractively low premiums but very skimpy benefits. A 2018 study by the Kaiser Family Foundation of two dozen short-term plans in 45 states found that 71 percent had no coverage for outpatient prescription drugs, 43 percent had no coverage for mental health services, and none covered maternity care. [5]

Here are some of the many examples across our health care system whereby quality of care is compromised by providers' quest for profits at the expense of patients.

1. Losing your insurance

This young man's only misfortune was having a 26th birthday, when he aged off his mother's ACA health insurance coverage:

> *Alec R. Smith had been on insulin for years for his Type 1 diabetes. He and his mother explored options over the three months before his birthday. His annual income as a restaurant manager was about $35,000, too high to qualify for Medicaid and also too high to be eligible for subsidies under Minnesota' ACA insurance marketplace. The plan they found [was unaffordable with] a monthly premium of $450 and an annual deductible of $7,600. He hoped to afford his $1,300 monthly bill for diabetes supplies [mostly for insulin, the cost of which had gone up by more than three-fold in the past seven years] by getting a part-time job. But he died of diabetic ketoacidosis a month later, just three days before payday, having apparently rationed his insulin, with an empty insulin syringe at his side.* [6]

Unfortunately, interruptions of health insurance are common and very hazardous for patients with Type I diabetes. A 2018 study found that one in four patients had at least one interruption over an average of 2.6 years, during which they needed many more acute care services, more ER visits, and hospitalizations. [7]

We know that health insurance for many Americans is unstable and volatile, whether by changes in networks or loss of Medicaid coverage in states with restrictive eligibility requirements. During these times of "churning," all of these previously insured are at higher vulnerability for complications and preventable deaths, especially those with chronic illnesses. It was estimated that the refusal by 20 states to expand Medicaid under the ACA would result in between 7,115 and 17,104 unnecessary deaths. [8]

2. Losing your doctor to insurer network changes

This is a common problem that disrupts continuity and quality of care for many patients and their families every year, usually with little advance notice. Refer back to Chapter 4, page 46, for Rasha Salama's experience as one such example. [9]

3. Skipping medications

According to the U. S. Centers for Disease Control and Prevention (CDC), almost 18 percent of working-age adults with diabetes are rationing their own medication by taking smaller doses, waiting to fill prescriptions, or skipping their treatments altogether. [10] This is not surprising, since the price of insulin has gone sky-high in recent years through blatant profiteering. A single vial of insulin now costs more than $250, and most patients use two to four vials each month. [11] With insulin so unaffordable, many patients are rationing insulin to the breaking point, including Alec Smith just mentioned and another Type I diabetic, Jesimya David Scherer-Radcliff, 21, who died more recently in rural Minnesota for the same reason. The two mothers comforted each other at Jesimya's memorial service saying "This is something we hoped would never happen again." [12]

The Boston area in Massachusetts has a booming economy in drug companies. One of these, Sanofi, has marked up its prices for insulin products by as much as 4,500 percent over the estimated cost of producing a single vial of insulin. As fatalities grow from rationing insulin, grieving mothers recently led a march against Sanofi, carrying the ashes of their dead children and demanding that the company cut its prices. [13]

4. Investor-owned care

If you still need confirmation of how widespread greed is throughout our system, with deleterious impacts on the quality of care of individual Americans and the population of this country, refer back to Table 3.1 on page 33 to summarize the disconnect that continues on unabated. The track record is clear and consistent for many years—corporate, investor-owned health care services cost much more and provide worse care than their not-for-profit counterparts.

5. Managed care by HMOs

Private health insurers have developed a bloated bureaucracy since the advent of managed care in the 1990s as they needed to set limits on referrals and hospitalizations, deny services, dis-enroll sick enrollees, and of course —to bill the payers. Remarkably, its workforce grew by one-third between 2000 and 2005, even as the overall health insurance market declined by one percent. [14] Overpayments are widespread to both privatized Medicare and Medicaid. Unnecessary or duplicative payments to Medicaid providers are common in more than 30 states. [15]

Malcolm Sparrow, author of the classic 2000 book, *License to Steal: How Fraud Bleeds America's Health Care System*, described the dark sides of the profit-driven managed care industry this way:

> *Under managed care, fraud will carry a much higher*
> *price in terms of human health. Fraud under managed*
> *care will claim lives. Testing will not be conducted when it*
> *should. Operations will not be performed when they should.*
> *Procedures will be carried out by inadequately qualified staff.*
> *Bureaucratic obstacles will be erected to deter patients from*
> *seeking treatment (and some patients will be deterred). Sick*
> *patients will be driven away.* [16]

6. Primary care shortage

Whereas generalist physicians, including family physicians, general internists and pediatricians, were the mainstay of our health care system in earlier years, it has become exceptional for patients and their families to have and keep such a physician on a continuity basis. Today, no more than 10 percent of U. S. medical graduates opt for family practice, while most internists and pediatricians move into subspecialties. The U. S. is facing a shortage of 52,000 primary care physicians by 2025. [17]

As a result of a near vacuum in primary care for first-contact and ongoing care of acute and chronic medical conditions, many patients seek care first at urgent care centers or emergency rooms, where they receive initial care without comprehensiveness, coordination or continuity of follow-up care. Patients today are ping-ponged around among specialists, whether in hospitals or as outpatients, often without adequate communication among them. The result is more fragmented and expensive care of lower quality for the majority of health conditions. As one common downside of this situation, polypharmacy is common among older adults who see multiple physicians, who don't talk to one another, for common problems. [18]

7. Medical errors

It is estimated that medical errors may account for more than 250,000 patient deaths a year in our fragmented system. [19] As one example, the ECRI Institute, a non-profit research group that studies patient safety, found that more than 7,600 so-called wrong-patient errors occurred at 181 health care organizations between 2013 and 2015. Most of these errors were caught before patients were harmed, but some were fatal, including one patient who was not resuscitated because of being confused with another patient who had a do-not-resuscitate order on file. [20]

8. Adverse drug reactions

These are still among the leading causes of hospitalization and deaths in this country, especially because of the fragmentation, discontinuity and lack of enough coordination of care.

II. Some Measures of Worse Outcomes of Care in the U. S.

Fortunately, we have an excellent organization in this country that has tracked the quality of U. S. health care for many years, both for comparisons with other advanced countries and U. S. state-by-state comparisons here—the Commonwealth Fund. It celebrated its centennial in 2018, having been founded by Anna Harkness in 1918 with the mandate to "do something for the welfare of mankind." Translated to health care, that means "to advance the common good by promoting a high-performing health care system that achieves better access, improved quality, and greater efficiency, particularly for society's most vulnerable, including low-income people, the uninsured, and people of color." [21] More than other resources, its website tells the story of U.S. health care over the last century, especially in terms of its accessibility, affordability, and quality of care.

Overall international measures

Figure 6.3 shows the extent to which older adults have greater cost barriers to care compared to ten other advanced countries. More than one-third of U. S. seniors have three or more chronic conditions and struggle to deal with high costs of care. Almost one-third of these patients skip care because of costs, compared to just 2 percent in Sweden, where universal coverage was enacted many years ago.[22]

A 2019 study comparing the U. S. and Canada concluded that socioeconomically vulnerable Canadians are consistently highly advantaged on health care access and outcomes through their single-payer system, and that the U. S. can expect that more than 50 million Americans will die earlier over the next generation unless it moves to a system of universal coverage. [23]

Figure 6.4 shows how poorly the U. S. does in terms of mortality amenable to health care compared to 15 other countries. Thomas Philippon, mentioned earlier, studied the health care systems in France, the U. K., Costa Rica, and the U. S. Figure 6.5 shows how France and the United Kingdom have far exceeded life expectancy in the U. S. since 2000, while the U. S. is on par with Costa Rica, a relatively less developed country.[24]

FIGURE 6.3

HIGH-NEED OLDER ADULTS EXPERIENCE GREATER COST BARRIERS TO RECEIVING CARE

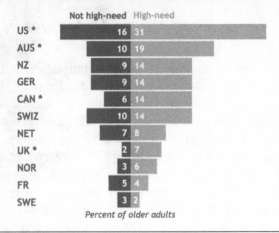

Percent of older adults

Source: 2017 The Commonwealth Fund International Health Policy Survey of Older Adults

FIGURE 6.4

CROSS NATIONAL COMPARISON OF MORTALITY AMENABLE TO HEALTH CARE

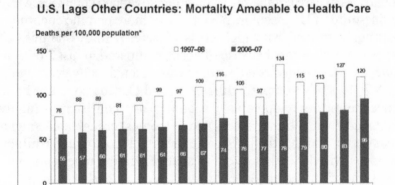

Source: Adapted from E. Nolte and M. McKee, "Variations in Amenable Mortality—Trends in 16 High-Income nations," *Health Policy,* published online Sept. 12, 2011

FIGURE 6.5

COMPARATIVE LIFE EXPECTANCY IN FOUR COUNTRIES

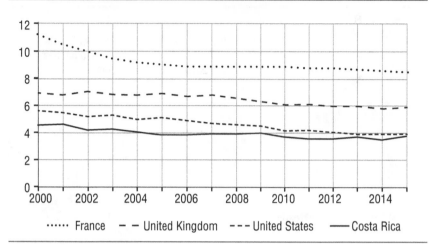

······ France   − − United Kingdom   - - - United States   —— Costa Rica

Source: Data Source OECD.

Overall state-by-state measures

The Commonwealth Fund has conducted studies of health care in all 50 states and the District of Columbia for almost ten years based on five measures—access and affordability, prevention and treatment, available hospital use and costs, healthy lives, and equity. Wide variations have been found from state to state and from region to region, as shown in Figure 6.6. [25]

Other measures
For-profit hospitals

Another measure of quality of care in this country compares for-profit hospitals with their not-for-profit counterparts in terms of re-admission rate over the 30 days after hospital discharge. Figure 6.7 shows that for-profit hospitals do less well for every medical condition for which patients were hospitalized.

FIGURE 6.6

OVERALL HEALTH SYSTEM PERFORMANCE

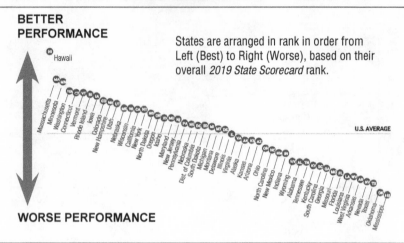

Source: The Commonwealth Fund, 2019

FIGURE 6.7

FOR-PROFIT HOSPITALS HAVE HIGHEST READMISSION RATES FOR **EVERY** CONDITION

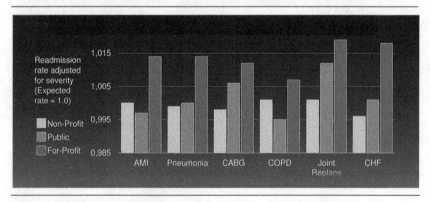

Source: PNHP, PLOS One 9/18/2018 - Based on Medicare Data

Nursing homes

About two-thirds of the nation's some 15,000 nursing homes are for-profit, many of which are in corporate chains. Their performance compared to not-for-profit counterparts has been studied for many years, with disturbing results that don't change. The for-profits have less nurses despite having sicker patients, as well as predictable worse quality of care and patient outcomes. The worst abusers are the largest corporate chains, such as Life Care Centers of America, now well-known for its being at the epicenter of the COVID-19 pandemic in Kirkland, Washington. It had eight deaths early on and a documented record of poor infectious disease protections as cited by federal regulators. [26]

This is what researchers have documented about these nursing home chains:

> *The chains have used strategies to maximize shareholder and investor value that include increasing Medicare revenues, occupancy rates, and company diversification, establishing multiple levels of corporate ownership, developing real estate trusts, and creating limited liability companies. These strategies enhance shareholder and investor profits, reduce corporate taxes, and reduce liability risk.* [27]

Over-utilization

It has been known for years that up to one-third of all health care services provided in the U. S. are unnecessary or inappropriate, with some actually harmful. [28] But this unaccountable practice goes on unabated, driven by a largely profit-oriented health care marketplace. A 2016 survey by the American Board of Internal Medicine found that three of four physicians surveyed believe that unnecessary tests and procedures are a serious problem. [29] Figure 6.8 helps to explain the dynamics of how over-utilization is a continuing problem. [30]

Prisons and mental health

Our system for mental health care is completely broken and underfunded. Many insurers exclude mental health services from their plans. Those that do cover them usually have inadequate numbers of psychiatrists and other mental health professionals in their networks. [31] Many psychiatrists and psychologists won't accept new patients with mental health problems, partly because of low reimbursement. Moreover, patients with psychoses and other serious mental health disorders often end up in jail, where many are seen as criminals and are not even treated for their problems.

FIGURE 6.8

PATHWAYS BY WHICH MORE MEDICAL CARE MAY LEAD TO HARM

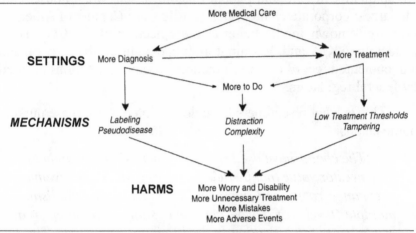

Source: Fisher, ES, Welch, HG. Avoiding the unintended consequences of growth in medical care: How might more be worse? *JAMA* 281:446-453, 1999.

The Mental Health Parity and Addiction Equity Act of 2008 was enacted to help level the playing field between medical/surgical services and mental health services, but it has been ineffective. The stigma of mental illness lives on, together with the lack of insurance coverage for mental health problems, as this family found out:

> *Joey Hudy started having delusions and paranoia in early 2017. His parents soon found that almost all of the possible treatment centers were out of network or out of state. They had to pay tens of thousands of dollars out-of-pocket to cover the costs of Joey's treatment, with no relief in sight.* [32]

III. What Can Be Done to Improve the Quality of Care?

Our current mostly private, complex multi-payer system is overly complex, bureaucratic, wasteful, and unsustainable as it profiteers on the backs of patients, their families, and taxpayers. Major reform is needed to improve quality of care in this country and start to compare better with all other advanced countries. These five steps will set a useful course toward that goal:

1. Recognize the failure of current and past attempts to improve quality

As is obvious, the "value-based" initiatives introduced by the ACA ten years ago have failed to improve quality of care in our profit-driven system. These include pay-for-performance (P4P) report cards for physicians and accountable care organizations, with some 150 quality metrics for outpatient services, such as for rates of screening mammography. Reporting on these puts an undue burden on physicians and staff, takes away many hours from patient care, and clearly hasn't worked. They are easily gamed through up-coding by billing clerks in hospitals and other facilities, thereby increasing their revenues but increasing costs to patients.

2. Financing reform—essential to better health care

The most important reform of all is to change how we finance health care. Corporate private health insurers have proven that their primary goal is to maximize revenues for their CEOs and shareholders at the expense of their enrollees. They have become disruptive to continuity of care and stand as barriers to quality as they limit care, deny services, and dis-enroll sicker enrollees. With administrative overhead at least five times higher than that of traditional public Medicare [33], they are themselves the elephant in the room.

We need to replace this multi-payer system with a new system of universal coverage through single-payer national health insurance (NHI), with equity for all based on medical need, not a privilege based on ability to pay. We should base this change on the principle that health care is not just another commodity for sale on an open marketplace, but instead is a human right that should be available to all Americans. Dr. Michael Fine, family physician and author of the 2018 book, *Health Care Revolt: How to Organize, Build a Health Care System, and Resuscitate Democracy—All at the Same Time*, gives us this challenge:

> *Health care is for people, not for profit. Insurance and markets are problems, not the solution. We need a health care system that cares for every American in every community.* [34]

3. Replace the current 'business ethic' with a largely not-for profit system and a strong service ethic

National polls since the 1970s have shown a long decline in the public's trust and respect for corporations, especially private insurers and the pharmaceutical industry, with only Congress and HMOs lower. [35] NHI can effectively shift toward a more service-oriented culture by implementing universal coverage and by price and cost controls through negotiated global budgets, bulk purchasing and other means.

4. Workforce planning, with increase for primary care, geriatrics, psychiatry, and public health

Well-performing health care systems in other advanced countries have a strong foundation of primary care that provides first-contact care; longitudinal continuity over time; comprehensiveness, with the capacity to diagnose and treat the majority of health problems; and coordination of care with other parts of the health care system. [36] Studies over many years have documented that primary care provides better health care for individuals and populations by improving access [37-39], containing costs [40], improving quality [41], and better coordination and integration of care.

We need to develop a national physician workforce plan that will address the growing shortage of primary care physicians, geriatricians, and psychiatrists, together with increased funding for public health.

5. Increased role of government

We cannot accomplish the above initiatives without a stronger role of government in several important areas—more effective planning, increased oversight and regulation, and science-based evaluation of treatments. The ACA took a limited approach to the latter need by establishing its Patient-Centered Outcomes Research Institute (PCORI), but it has been underfunded, subject to undue industry influence, and even banned from using cost-effectiveness or quality-adjusted life years (QALYs) in its recommendations. [42]

Josepth Stiglitz, Ph.D., Nobel Laureate in Economics and former chief economist at the World Bank, called for a larger role of government in this way in 2004:

> *Markets do not lead to efficient outcomes, let alone outcomes that comport with social justice. As a result, there is often good reason for government intervention to improve the efficiency of the market. Just as the Great Depression should have made it evident that the market does not work as well as its advocates claim, our Roaring Nineties should have made it self-evident that the pursuit of self-interest does not necessarily lead to overall economic efficiency.* [43]

Conclusion:

Who is our system for? We need to answer this urgent moral question. In the last chapter we'll consider whether we're up to that. The insulin story is a tragic example of the kind of greed-driven health care system that we have. Many more examples will be discussed across the medical-industrial complex in Chapter 9, including the role that corruption and fraud play into this Achilles heel of American health care. But for now, let's move to the next chapter to describe another related problem that adversely impacts our population—the increasing inequality and disparities within our society.

References:

1.   Caper, P. The ills of money-driven medicine. Op-Ed, *Bangor Daily News*, May 21, 2012.
2.   Belluz, J. Thousands of heart patients get stents that may do more harm than good. *Vox*, November 6, 2017.
3.   Philippon, T. *The Great Reversal: How America Gave Up on Free Markets* Cambridge, MA. *The Belknap Press of Harvard University*, 2019, pp. 223-224.
4.   Saad, L. More Americans delaying medical treatment due to cost, *Gallup*, December 9, 2019.
5.   Cunningham, PW, Firozi, P. The health care world slams Trump's proposal for short-term plans. *The Washington Post*, April 24, 2018.
6.   Sable-Smith, B. Insulin's high cost leads to lethal rationing. *NPR*, September 1, 2018.

7. Rogers, MAM, Lee, JM, Tipirneni, R et al. Interruptions in private health insurance and outcomes in adults with Type I diabetes: A longitudinal study. *Health Affairs*, July 2018.
8. Dickman, S et al. Opting out of Medicaid expansion: The health and financial impacts. *Health Affairs Blog*, January 30, 2014.
9. Galewitz, P. Needy patients 'caught in the middle' as insurance titan drops doctors. *Kaiser Health News*, February 25, 2020.
10. Cohn, J. Health care rationing? It's already reality under private insurance. *The Progressive Populist*, September 15, 2019.
11. Altman, D. It's not just the uninsured—it's also the cost of health care. *Axios,* August 20, 2018.
12. Ibid # 10.
13. Saini, V. As drug prices rise, is Boston's prosperity based on a moral crime. *WBUR*, January 31, 2019.
14. Herman, B. Medicaid's unmanaged managed care. *Modern Healthcare*, April 30, 2016.
15. *National Health Expenditure Data—Historical*. Centers for Medicare and Medicaid Services.
16. Sparrow, MK. *License to Steal: How Fraud Bleeds America's Health Care System*. Boulder, CO. *Westview Press*, 2000, p. 112.
17. Peterson, SM, Liaw, WR, Phillips, RL et al. Projecting U. S. primary care physician workforce needs: 2010-2025. *Ann Fam Med* 10 (6): 503-509, 2012.
18. Landro, L. Medication overload. *Wall Street Journal*, October 1, 2016: D1.
19. Bakalar, N. Medical errors may cause over 250,000 deaths a year. *New York Times*, May 3, 2016.
20. Beck, M. Wrong-patient errors called common. *Wall Street Journal*, September 26, 2016: A 2.
21. Mission statement of the Commonwealth Fund, *The Commonwealth Centennial*, May 31, 2018.
22. Osborn, R, Doty, MM, Moulds, D et al. Older Americans were sicker and faced more financial barriers to health care than counterparts in other countries. 2017 Commonwealth Fund International Health Policy Survey of Older Adults, November 15, 2017. New York. *Commonwealth Fund*.
23. Escobar, KM, Murariu, D, Munro, S. Care of acute conditions and chronic diseases in Canada and the United States: Rapid systemic review and meta-analysis. *J Public Health Research*, March 11, 2019.
24. Ibid # 3, p. 224-225.
25. CWF State by State Scorecard, 2019. *The Commonwealth Fund.*
26. Harrington, C, Houser, C, Olney, B et al. Ownership, financing and management strategies of the ten largest nursing home chains in the United States. *Intl J Health Services* 41 (4): 725-746, 2011.
27. Read, R. Welcome to the U. S. coronavirus epicenter. Stores are empty and firefighters in quarantine as the death toll rises in Kirkland, WA. *Los Angeles Times*, March 5, 2010.
28. Wenner, JB, Fisher, ES. Skinner, JS. Geography and the debate over Medicare reform. *Health Affairs Web Exclusive* W-103, February 13, 2002.

29. Hancock, J. How tiny are benefits from many tests and pills? Researchers paint a picture. *Kaiser Health News*, October 12, 2016.
30. Fisher, ES, Welch, HG. Avoiding the unintended consequences of growth in medical care: How might more be worse? *JAMA* 281: 446-453, 1999.
31. Andrews, M. Narrow networks get even tighter when shopping for mental health specialists. *Kaiser Health News*, September 22, 2017.
32. Kennedy, PJ. Insurance system still discriminates against mental illness. *USA Today*, October 3, 2018.
33. Frakt, A. *Private vs. Public Prices. Academy Health Blog*, January 13, 2017.
34. Fine, M. *Health Care Revolt: How to Organize, Build a Health Care System, and Resuscitate Democracy—All at the Same Time.* Oakland, CA. *PM Press*, 2018, p. 138.
35. Patashnik, E. Why American doctors keep doing expensive procedures that don't work. *VOX*, February 14, 2018.
36. Starfield, B. Is primary care essential? *The Lancet* 344 (8930): 1129-1133, 1994.
37. Parchman, ML, Culler, S. Primary care physicians and avoidable hospitalization. *J Fam Pract* 39: 122-128, 1994.
38. Greenfield, S, Nelson, EC, Zubkoff, M et al. Variations in resource utilization among medical specialties and systems of care: Results from the Medical Outcomes Study. *JAMA* 267 (12): 1624-1630, 1992.
39. Ferrante, Gonzales, EC, Pal, N et al. Effects of physician supply on early detection of breast cancer. *J Am Board of Fam Pract* 13: 408-414, 2000.
40. Franks, P, Fiscella, K. Primary care physicians and specialists as personal physicians: health care expenditures and mortality experience. *J Fam Pract* 47: 103-104, 1998.
41. Roetzheim, RG, Pal, N, Gonzales, EC et al. The effects of physician supply on the early detection of colorectal cancer. *J Fam Pract* 48 (11): 850-858, 1999.
42. Gerber, AS, Patashnik, EM, Doherty, D et al. The public wants information, not board mandates, from comparative effectiveness research. *Health Affairs* 29 (10): 1879, 2010.
43. Stiglitz, JE. Evaluating economic change. *Daedalus* 133/3, Summer 2004.

Chapter 7

INCREASING HEALTH DISPARITIES AND INEQUITIES

We're used to thinking of a depression as geographic, but this one is demographic. Working class Americans, often defined as those without a college degree, are caught in a dust bowl. . . . It is these working class Americans, white and black alike, who have seen earnings collapse, family structure disintegrate and mortality climb. These Americans are earning less on average, adjusted for inflation, than their counterparts back in the 1970s. . . . The central fact of America today is not its economic vigor but its profound inequity. [1]

—Nicholas Kristof, two-time Pulitzer Prize winning journalist and co-author of the 2020 book, *Tightrope: Americans Reaching for Hope.*

As pointed out so clearly by Nicholas Kristof above, inequality and inequities have increased exponentially over the last 50 years so as to threaten the cohesion of American society. The extent of this change is mind-boggling: average income for the top 1 % has risen by $800,000 since 1970; for the top 0.1 %, by $4 million; for the top .01 %, by $20 million, all while the average income for the bottom 50 % of Americans has gone up by just $8,000. [2] A poll conducted by the Pew Research Center in 2014 found that a plurality ranked inequality as the "greatest danger in the world," above that of "religious and ethnic hatred," nuclear weapons, and environmental degradation. [3]

The goals of this chapter are three-fold: (1) to bring some historical perspective to disparities and inequities in American society over the years; (2) to show how they impact health care for individuals and populations across the country; and (3) to briefly consider two major approaches that can go a long way to redress these adverse impacts.

I. Historical Perspective on Disparities and Inequities in the U. S.

Inequality within the U. S. population has been steadily increasing for many years, while disparities in health care are multi-dimensional, based on such factors as socioeconomic status, race/ethnicity, age, gender, location, and disability status. Today, the richest 0.1 percent in the U. S. control a bigger share of the pie than at any time since 1929. [4] Figure 7.1 gives us a graphic picture of how this has come about since 1910 in this country. [5]

FIGURE 7.1

THE UPSURGE IN U.S. WEALTH INEQUALITY

(Top 1% and bottom 90% shares of total private US wealth)

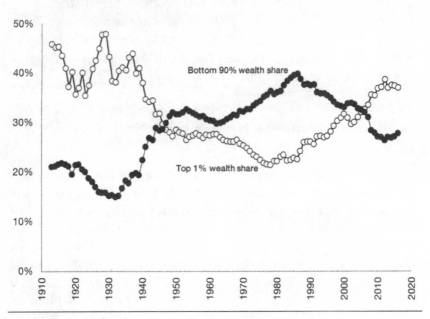

Source: Saez, E, Zucman, G. *The Triumph of Injustice: How the Rich Dodge Taxes and How to Make Them Pay.* New York. *W. W. Norton & Company,* 2019, p. 98.

Both income and wealth disparities have grown enormously over these years. Bringing all this up to today, the bottom 90 percent of Americans average an annual income today of about $30,000 compared to the annual incomes of the top 0.01 percent of $35 million.

Jim Hightower of the *Hightower Lowdown* breaks down this uninterrupted trend for growing income and wealth disparities with these startling statistics:

- "One in five Americans has zero net worth. Or less. Many of us owe more than we own and, living paycheck to paycheck, can't get ahead to build a nest egg.
- U. S. wealth disparity is the greatest of any advanced economy in the world, with the richest 1 % holding more of our nation's wealth than the bottom 90 % of us!
- Just three Americans—Jeff Bezos (Amazon), Bill Gates (Microsoft), and Warren Buffett (Berkshire-Hathaway)— possess more personal wealth ($248 billion) than the entire bottom half. Yes, more than 165 million of us combined." [6]

As Hightower observes:

The rapidly widening divide between the rich and the rest of us is neither natural nor accidental. During the past half century, myriad corporate and governmental decisions— from labor law to campaign finance regulations—have methodically slanted America's economic and political systems so that money and power flow from the many to the few. The plutocrats' most effective and least reported-on-tool is America's tax structure. . . Multimillionaires and billionaires don't usually draw the bulk of their fabulous incomes from paychecks, but from their enormous financial assets, i.e., their wealth. This inherited or accumulated wealth generates "capital income"—and further wealth—with little or no work by the asset holder. [7]

The Center for American Progress, in a 2019 report concluded that the moral basis of U. S. tax policy has been perverted since the 1980s by legislative and regulatory twists that tax work, but leave the huge accumulations of wealth virtually avoiding taxation. [8] Meanwhile, the bottom 90 percent now pay almost as much in taxes as the top 0.1 percent, as shown in Figure 7.2, which also shows that the average tax rate for the rich was 55 percent during the Eisenhower administration. [9]

FIGURE 7.2

THE AVERAGE TAX RATE FOR THE RICH UNDER EISENHOWER—55%

(Average tax rates: top 0.1% versus bottom 90% income earners)

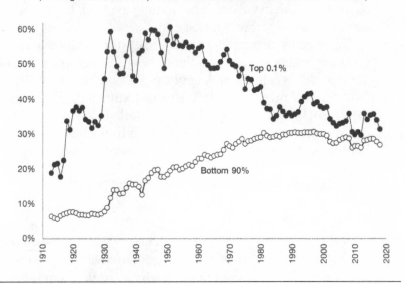

Source: Saez, E, Zucman, G. *The Triumph of Injustice: How the Rich Dodge Taxes and How to Make Them Pay.* New York. *W. W. Norton & Company*, 2019, p. 42.

President Barack Obama, in his farewell address to Congress in January, 2017, called inequality the "defining challenge of our time." [10] Unfortunately, however, he didn't do much about it during his eight years in office. Economic inequality grew rapidly despite strong economic indicators, with almost all of the new income since the Great Recession going to the top 1 percent. He also supported extension of the Bush tax cuts on the wealthy in 2010. [11]

These examples illustrate the extreme polar opposites in today's society, with little communication or understanding between the two. On the one hand, millennials near middle age are in crisis. Fewer get married, have kids, own a home, and graduate from college; they also have lower household net worth. [12] On the other hand, Jeff Bezos of Amazon, the wealthiest American, just purchased the most expensive residential property in the history of Los Angeles for $165 million, less than 1 percent of his $131.9 billion net worth. This at the same time that the U. S. set a new record for the highest number of homeless school kids in modern history. Trump's proposed 2021 budget proposal fuels further inequality, with deep cuts to Medicare,

Medicaid and Social Security, despite his previous promises not to cut them. [13]

How can we explain this 50-year history of such radical change in what it is to be an American? In his thoughtful recent article in *The New Yorker*, Joshua Rothman makes this useful observation that helps to describe the ongoing unresolved tension between the haves and have nots: "As Americans we are charged with recognizing two conflicting values: individualism and egalitarianism." [14] As we are increasingly being pulled apart, it seems that egalitarianism is losing out, and that we need to start pulling together, especially in a time of a coronavirus pandemic and a major recession. Robert Reich, Professor of Public Policy at the University of California Berkeley's Goldman School of Public Policy and author of 15 books, including *The Common Good* and *Saving Capitalism,* brings us a vision of how to do this:

> *The common good consists of our shared values about what we owe one another as citizens who are bound together in the same society—the norms we voluntarily abide by, and the ideals we seek to achieve. . . A concern for the common good—keeping the common good in mind—is a moral attitude. It recognizes that we're all in it together. If there is no common good, there is no society.* [15]

That direction is especially important as we next look at disparities and inequities in health care.

II. How Disparities and Inequities Impact U. S. Health Care

As disparities and inequities grow and as our population becomes more heterogeneous, many more Americans are vulnerable in our dysfunctional, profit-driven health care system. With less access to affordable care, disadvantaged groups have a higher burden of illness, injury, disability and mortality compared to their more advantaged counterparts. As one example, low-income adults in Alabama are almost seven times more likely than high-income people to skip needed care because of cost. [16]

Stereotypes and stigmas, such as racism, sexism, ageism, and attitudes toward the disabled or mentally ill, create further access barriers to necessary care. Figure 7.3 shows how discrimination in health care predicts further disability. [17]

FIGURE 7.3

DISCRIMINATION IN HEALTH CARE
PREDICTS NEW DISABILITY

A Prospective Study of Older Adults

Percent with worsening disability over next 4 years

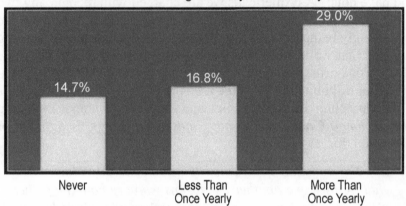

| Never | Less Than Once Yearly | More Than Once Yearly |

How Frequently Do You Experience Discrimination in Care?

Source: Rogers, SE, Thrasher, AD, Miao, Y et al. Discrimination in health care settings is associated with disability in older adults: Health and retirement study, 2008-2012. *J Gen Intern Med* 30 (10): 1413-1420, 2015.

Let's look at seven major factors that contribute to restricted access to essential care and worse outcomes.

1. Socioeconomic determinants

Although the ACA did bring some temporary improvement in access to care, it remains unaffordable for much of our population as disparities continue unabated. A 2013 report from the Institute of Medicine (now the National Academy of Medicine), noted that today's measures of quality of care fail to account for socioeconomic factors:

> *Adverse social and economic conditions also matter greatly to health and affect a large segment of the U. S. population. Despite its large and powerful economy, the United States has higher rates of poverty and income inequality than most high-income countries. U. S. children are more likely than children in peer countries to grow up in poverty, and the proportion of today's children who will improve their*

*socioeconomic position and earn more than their parents
is smaller than in many other high-income countries. . .
Finally, Americans have less access to the kinds of 'safety net'
programs that help buffer the effects of adverse economic and
social conditions in other countries.* [18]

According to the Commonwealth Fund's cross-national studies of health care in eleven advanced countries, the U. S. lags significantly behind all ten other countries in life expectancy. Roosa Tikkanen, a research associate there, summed it up this way: "We live sicker and die younger than our counterparts around the world."[19]

2. Poverty

In this land of supposed plenty, there are 43 million Americans living in poverty out of our population of 326 million. [20] The Trump administration and Republicans in Congress are working, under the guise of "welfare reform," to make the plight of poor and low-income people worse through cuts to Medicaid and other safety net programs. Not stopping there, they are also giving out more waivers to states to further restrict eligibility for Medicaid and even to re-define poverty itself. Trump has proposed shifting to a so-called "chained CPI," which would slow the pace of price gains more than measures used since the 1960s, thereby recalculating the federal poverty level lower and limiting eligibility for Medicaid. [21] Even beyond that, through its "public charge rules," lawful immigration can now be denied when families seek or obtain nutrition assistance, housing, or health care for which they qualify. Now, for the first time in decades, U. S. citizen children with immigrant parents are almost four times as likely to lose Medicaid coverage than those with native-born parents. [22]

3. Lack of insurance coverage

Here is what it means for real people to be uninsured in this country with such a supposedly excellent health care system.

*Sarai was born with Wilson's disease, an inherited
disorder that leads to liver failure. She could have been cured
by having a liver transplant, but was denied at two prominent
liver transplant hospitals in Chicago for lack of insurance
coverage. She died at age 25, when her physician signed her*

death certificate as liver failure. The real cause of her death, however, was inequality. [23]

Larry Churchill, Ph.D., well-known ethicist at the University of Notre Dame, is spot-on with his reaction to this kind of care:

A health system which neglects the poor and disenfranchised impoverishes the social order of which we all are constituted. In a real (and not just hortatory) sense, a health care system is no better than the least well-served of its members. [24]

In a recent historical review trying to answer the question why the U. S. has never come around to universal health care, Jeneen Interlandi, a member of the Editorial Board for *The New York Times,* builds a persuasive case that the answer has everything to do with racism. She recounts how African-Americans, at the close of the Civil War, had a considerably higher mortality rate from smallpox. In non-response, white leaders feared black epidemics spilling over into their own communities. As a result, they deployed few physicians to the war-torn South, ignored their pleas for help, and prematurely shut down hospitals. One hundred and fifty years after the freed people of the South first petitioned the government for basic medical care, the U. S. remains an outlier as the only high-income country in the world without universal access to health care.[25]

Evelynn Hammonds, an historian of science at Harvard University, sums up the situation this way:

There has never been any period in American history where the health of blacks was equal to that of whites. Disparity is built into the system. [26]

Although Medicare, Medicaid and the ACA have helped to ameliorate some of these disparities, we still are far from a system of universal access to health care. Without universal coverage, the Trump administration's immigration policy, with its new "public charge" rule, will exacerbate the spread of coronavirus by deterring millions of non-citizens, for fear of imperiling their immigration status, from seeking medical care through such safety net programs as Medicaid. [27]

Now enter the coronavirus pandemic, and physicians in public health and on the front lines are reporting familiar patterns of racial and economic bias in response to it. Examples include drive-through testing centers being located in more affluent white neighborhoods, together with delayed diagnosis and treatment for people of color. The impact of these inequities are not yet well known since the CDC does not report data on race and states' reports are only fragmentary.[28] But we already know that an increasing number of cities are reporting large disparities in deaths from COVID-19, such as in Chicago, where African-Americans represent 30 percent of the population but account for more than 70 percent of these deaths. [29]

Jeneen Interlandi recently tweeted this important observation:

Our society is constructed to reward the rich in good times and punish the poor in bad times. A coronavirus recession would be doubly painful, as lower-income households are likely to pay a heavier toll in both health and wealth. [30]

4. Ageism

While a multi-generational workforce is becoming the norm in the U. S., with more than 117 million people over age 50 working, age discrimination in the workplace and in health care is a significant problem. A new AARP study conducted by the Economist Intelligence Unit has documented growing workplace practices that discriminate against older people, including involuntary retirement, under employment, and unemployment, as shown in Figure 7.4. [31]

Here is a humorous, but also serious example of how older patients are frequently insensitively disregarded by physicians without much concern:

A 97-year-old man goes to his doctor with a painful left knee, without any history of a fall or other trauma. After examining the knee, the doctor dismissively says: "Hey, the knee is 97 years old, what do you expect?" The patient replies: But my right knee is 97 and doesn't hurt a bit! [32]

FIGURE 7.4

THE REAL COST
OF DISCRIMINATION

The U.S. missed out on
$850 billion in economic
activity in 2018 due to biases
against older workers. Here's
what the amount is attributed to:

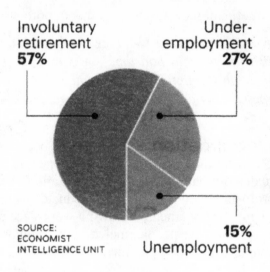

Involuntary
retirement
57%

Under-
employment
27%

SOURCE:
ECONOMIST
INTELLIGENCE UNIT

15%
Unemployment

Source: AARP , March 2020

5. *Women's health care*

An escalating war on women has been waged by conservative
Republicans and the Trump administration targeting women's
reproductive rights. These efforts have included restricting the Title
X Family Planning Program enacted during the Nixon administration
in 1970 and intention to overturn the 1973 Roe v. Wade Supreme
Court decision allowing abortion. Their efforts have succeeded in
defunding much of Title X, with closure of family planning clinics
in many states, and moving Roe v. Wade to a future hearing by the
U. S. Supreme Court.

Unfortunately, many American women have paid a high cost
for removal of these services and protections. Sixty-one million are

at risk of unintended pregnancy during their childbearing years (15 to 44). In order to avoid an undesired pregnancy during those years, they have to depend on contraceptive use for about three decades. Couples not using contraceptives are at about an 85 percent risk of an unintended pregnancy. Improved birth control and access to family planning clinics led to reduction of the U. S. abortion rate to a new low in 2014. The Guttmacher Institute calls attention to the importance of contraceptive use in these compelling words:

> *The ability to delay and space childbearing is crucial to women's social and economic advancement. Women's ability to obtain and effectively use contraceptives has a positive impact on their education and workforce participation, as well as on subsequent outcomes related to income, family stability, mental health and happiness, and children's well being.* [33]

Opponents of family planning clinics fail to recognize that 97 percent of Planned Parenthood family planning services are for preventive services, including breast exams, screening for cervical cancer and sexually transmitted infections, with only 3 percent for abortion. [34] The hypocrisy of opponents to these services is shown by this statement by Dr. Hal Lawrence, CEO of the American College of Obstetricians and Gynecologists:

> *The strange thing about this is that people who want to decrease the number of abortions are taking away access to the very services that help prevent them.* [35]

Meanwhile, as conservatives continue their battle against women's health care, we are # 46 in the world in maternal death rates among developed nations, with between 700 and 900 women dying preventable deaths each year from causes related to pregnancy or childbirth. [36]

6. Mental health care

Stigma concerning mental health problems has been a long-standing problem in our culture, which values physical problems above mental health disorders. Although the Mental Health Parity Act and Addiction Equity Act was enacted in 2008 requiring health plans to cover mental health services at least as generously as for medical/surgical services, the stigma and restricted access to care remains.

Almost one in five Americans has had some kind of mental illness or addiction disorder in the past year. Barriers to care include poor insurance coverage, narrow networks, shortage of psychiatrists and psychologists, and low reimbursement for mental health services. [37] Many patients who cannot gain access to care end up in jail, where they are criminalized and often left untreated. A national survey of county jails by Public Citizen's Health Research Group drew this conclusion in 2016:

> *This growing problem is not solely a criminal justice problem. At its heart is evidence of the unacceptable failure of our public mental health system.* [38]

7. Rural health care

Residents of America's rural areas comprise another major group of our population that is disadvantaged by growing inequities within our profit-driven system. Rural hospitals are the hub of accessible health care, and often are the largest employer in the community. But they are under-reimbursed, and have been hit hard by funding cuts, especially from Medicaid. Since 2010, 106 rural hospitals have closed across the country, with another 430—or 1 in 5 remaining—at high risk of closure. [39]

When rural hospitals close, rural residents are left without adequate care, especially for trauma, maternity care, and other urgent and emergent medical problems that then require long trips to the nearest hospital to get care. Other parts of the rural health crisis include the closure of nursing homes and pharmacies (often triggered by corporate decisions that they are not sufficiently profitable to be continued), shortages of physicians and other health professionals, and the aging of rural populations that need more care, not less. [40, 41]

To the above list of inequities, of course, we need to add the worse care and outcomes of enrollees in privatized Medicare and Medicaid, as dealt with in earlier chapters.

III. Approaches to Reduce These Adverse Impacts on Health Care

We have to ask whether the playing field can be leveled to grant needed access to affordable health care for our entire population. Joseph Stiglitz, Ph.D., Nobel Laureate in Economics and former chief economist at the World Bank, has concluded that the overall problem is that we have been pursuing a trickle-down economic policy that benefits the 1 percent, not the rest of us. [42]

Here are two basic approaches that can provide the framework for other enabling steps to redress disparities and inequities.

1. Tax reform

In the debate over our future in the current 2020 election cycle, major tax reform is being called for, especially by progressive candidates. Senator Elizabeth Warren proposed an annual 2 percent tax on assets of $50 million and a 3 percent tax on assets above $1 billion. [43] As she said during her presidential campaign:

> *There's nobody in this country who got rich on their own—nobody. You built a factory out there? Good for you! But I want to be clear: You moved your goods to market on the roads the rest of us paid for. You hired workers the rest of us paid to educate. You were safe in your factory because of police forces and fire forces the rest of us paid for. You built a factory and it turned into something terrific . . . God bless! Keep a hunk of it. But part of the underlying social contract is you take a hunk of that and pay it forward to the next kid who comes along.* [44]

2. Universal coverage

Responding to the GOP and Trump administration's ongoing attack against Medicaid, Michael Corcoran of *Truthout* draws this important conclusion, based on long experience in this country:

> *Until the Unites States adopts a model of social insurance that provides health care to all, regardless of income, the poor will continue to be treated like collateral damage in the war against equality and justice.* [45]

Conclusion

We will discuss these and other approaches to health care reform in some detail in Chapter 11, but for now we need to turn to the next chapter, where we will describe the extent to which profiteering, corruption, and even fraud undermine the goals of any good health care system and continue to block real reform.

References:

1. Kristof, ND. Part of America is still forgotten, now under Trump. *Seattle Times*, February 8, 2020.
2. Conley, J. 'Staggering' new data show income of top 1% has grown 100 times faster than bottom 50% since 1970. *Common Dreams*, December 9, 2019.
3. Pew Research Center, as cited by Rothman, J. Same difference. What the idea of equality can do for us, and what it can't. *The New Yorker*, January 13, 2020.
4. Johnson, J. World's 500 richest people gained $1.2 trillion in wealth in 2019: Analysis. *Common Dreams*, December 27, 2019.
5. Saez, E, Zucman, G. *The Triumph of Injustice: How the Rich Dodge Taxes and How to Make Them Pay*. New York. *W. W. Norton & Company*, 2019, p. 98.
6. Hightower, J. It's time for a (teeny) tax on Wealth. *The Hightower Lowdown* 21 (8): 1-2, September 2019.
7. Ibid # 6.
8. Center for American Progress. June 2019 report.
9. Ibid # 5, p. 42.
10. Carter, Z. *Politics*, January 11, 2017.) (Complete ref)
11. Hoxie, J. Obama's take on inequality. *Institute for Policy Studies Program on Inequality and the Common Good*, January 13, 2017.
12. Adamy, J, Overberg, P. Millennials near middle age in crisis. *Wall Street Journal,* May 20, 2019: A1.
13. Benjamin, R. Trump's 2021 budget fuel inequality. *Los Angeles Times*, February 21, 2020.
14. Rothman, J. Same difference. What the idea of equality can do for us, and what it can't. *The New Yorker*, January 13, 2020.
15. Reich, RB. *The Common Good*. New York. *Alfred A Knopf*, 2018, p. 18.
16. 2018 Scorecard on State Health System Performance. New York. *The Commonwealth Fund.*

17. Rogers, SE, Thrasher, AD, Miao, Y et al. Discrimination in health care settings is associated with disability in older adults: Health and retirement study, 2008-2012. *J Gen Intern Med* 30 (10): 1413-1420, 2015.

18. Woolf, SH, Aron, L (eds). *U. S. Health in International Perspective: Shorter Lives, Poorer Health.* National Research Council. Institute of Medicine. Washington, D.C. *The National Academies Press,* 2013.

19. Tikkanen, R. As quoted by Pizzigati, S. Living in inequality, dying in despair. *The Progressive Populist,* March 15, 2020, p. 10.

20. Powers, N. Fear of a black planet: Under the Republican push for welfare cuts, racism boils. *Truthout,* January 21, 2018.

21. Sink, J. Trump may redefine poverty, cutting Americans from welfare rolls. *Bloomberg.* May 6, 2019.

22. Dorn, S and R. Collateral damage: The administration's public charge immigration restrictions are endangering health coverage for U. S. citizen children. *Families USA,* February 21, 2020.

23. Ansell, D. I watched my patients die of poverty for 40 years. It's time for single payer. *The Washington Post,* September 13, 2017.

24. Churchill, LR. *Rationing Health Care in America: Perceptions and Principles of Justice.* Notre Dame, Ind. *University of Notre Dame,* 1987, p. 103.

25. Interlandi, J. Why doesn't the United States have universal health care? The answer has everything to do with race. *New York Times,* August 14, 2019.

26. Hammonds, E. As quoted by Ibid # 25.

27. The Editorial Board. With coronavirus, 'health care for some' is a recipe for disaster. *New York Times,* March 6, 2020.

28. Farmer, B. Long-standing racial and income disparities seen creeping into COVID-19 care. *Modern Healthcare,* April 6, 2020.

29. African Americans comprise more than 70% of COVID-19 deaths in Chicago, officials say. *CBS News,* April 6, 2020

30. Interlandi, J. Twitter, March 10, 2020.

31. Jenkins, JA. Age bias costs us all. *AARP Bulletin,* March 2020: 38.

32. Graham, J. A doctor speaks out about ageism in medicine. *Kaiser Health News,* May 30, 2019.

33. Dreweke, J. Anti-choice Republicans likely to ignore key reason for abortion rate decline. *Guttmacher Institute,* January 17, 2017.

34. Alonzo-Zalvidar, R, Crary, D. Trump remaking federal policy on women's reproductive health. *Associated Press,* May 30, 2018

35. Lawrence, H. As quoted in Corbett, J. 'Crisis no one is talking about': GOP threatens health care of 26 million people. *Common Dreams,* February 2, 2018.

36. West, E. Why single-payer is a feminist issue. *Truthout,* January 21, 2018.

37. Andrews, M. Narrow networks get even tighter when shopping for mental health specialists. *Kaiser Health News,* September 22, 2017.

38. Bradberry, A, Goodwin, D. National survey shows county jails unequipped, overwhelmed with seriously mentally ill inmates. *Public Citizen News,* September/October 2016, p. 4.

39. Heitkamp, H. America's rural health care crisis must be addressed. *Heidi Heitkamp*, June 12, 2019.
40. Healy, J. Nursing homes are closing across rural America, scattering residents. *New York Times*, March 4, 2019.
41. Langreth, R, Ingold, D, Gu, J. Secret drug pricing system middlemen use to rake in millions. *Bloomberg*, September 11, 2018.
42. Stiglitz, J. *The Price of Inequality*. New York. *Penguin*, 2013.
43. Johnson, J. World's 500 richest people gained $1 trillion in wealth in 2019: Analysis. *Common Dreams*, December 27, 2019.
44. Warren, E, as quoted by Hightower, Ibid # 6, p. 3.
45. Corcoran, M. A legal battle is mounting against the GOP's attack on Medicaid. *Truthout*, February 6, 2018.

PART III

CORRUPTION AND FRAUD ACROSS THE MEDICAL - INDUSTRIAL COMPLEX

So it is that contrary to what we have heard rhetorically for a generation now, the individualist, greed-driven, free market ideology is at odds with our history and with what most Americans really care about. More and more people agree that growing inequality is bad for the country, that corporations have too much power, that money in politics is corrupting democracy and that working and poor communities need and deserve help when the market system fails to generate shared prosperity. Indeed, the American public is committed to a set of values that almost perfectly contradicts the conservative agenda that has dominated politics for a generation now. [1]

—Bill Moyers [1]

Nothing about monopolization is inevitable. Our increasingly dystopian and corrupt apparatus was brought to us by people selling a fantasy of inevitability. Some of them sold us a right-wing fantasy of corporate monopolies and bigness as a sign of progress. Some of them sold us a left-wing fantasy of corporate monopolies as an unstoppable feature of capitalism. But these fantasies are, in the end, the same. They both are designed to sell you on the idea that you have no power, that you are nothing but a consumer.

And that is not true. It never has been true. America has always been a nation of tradespeople. We embed social justice in our banks, our corporations, our markets, in how we exchange goods, services, crops, ideas, and labor with one another. Each of us is a worker, a business person, a consumer, and a citizen. The real question is not whether commerce is good or bad. It is how we are to do commerce, to serve concentrated power or to free ourselves from concentrated power. . . . The truth is, America is a battle, a struggle for justice. And we choose, every generation, who wins. [2]

—Matt Stoller, author of *Goliath: The 100-Year War Between Monopoly Power and Democracy*

(1). Moyers, B. A New Story for America. *The Nation* 284 (3): 17, 2007.
(2) Stoller, M. *Goliath: The 100-Year War Between Monopoly Power and Democracy*. New York. *Simon & Schuster*, 2019, p. 456.

Chapter 8

RUNAWAY PROFITEERING, CORRUPTION, FRAUD AND WASTE

Our health care system has been driven largely by profit, rather than by measures of health. Countless providers, companies, consultants and intermediaries are trying to get their piece of the $3.5 trillion pie that is U. S. health care. In 21st century U. S. health care, everything is revenue, and so everything is billed. [1]

—Dr. Elizabeth Rosenthal, ER physician, editor-in-chief of *Kaiser Health News*, and author of *An American Sickness: How Healthcare Became Big Business and How You Can Take It Back*

As we saw in the last three chapters, our dysfunctional, profit-driven health care system, with its soaring prices and costs, results in decreased access to care, worse quality, and increasing disparities and inequities. In this chapter, we will look more closely across the medical-industrial complex to tease out four big contributors to this overall problem—profiteering, corruption, fraud and waste. They are intertwined and tend to bleed into each other, to the point where some fraud doesn't actually break the law. As we proceed, you can make your own decision as to which is which!

So this chapter has three goals: (1) to give a brief overview of the cost problem and a comparison to other advanced countries; (2) to describe the extent of profiteering, corruption and fraud across various parts of our system; and (3) to briefly consider the cumulative extent of waste from all these excesses that exacerbates the costs that patients have to pay in order to receive care in this country.

I. Overall picture

To get started, consider a recent blog by Bob Laszewski, president of Health Policy and Strategy Associates, a Washington D.C. based policy and marketplace consulting firm. He has been named a "Top Speaker" on health care in a survey involving 13,000 business leaders, educators and others. Here are some excerpts from his early 2020 blog, entitled Profitability in the Health Care Market Has Never Been Better, that focuses on the state of Florida, but which he feels is also representative of other states across the country:

- "Continued expansion by health insurers and hospitals systems combined with coverage expansion has improved profits for both. Profits for Florida HMOs increased by 12% in 2018. . .
- The health insurance market has grown significantly more concentrated in the last three years as companies like Anthem and Blue Cross Blue Shield have acquired a number of HMOs. . .
- As a result of their market power and favorable claims experience, HMOs enjoyed strong profits in 2018, particularly on their individual and Medicare Advantage plans. Florida HMOs had net income of just under $1 billion in 2018. . .
- Individual market health insurers finally figured out how to make money on Obamacare (ACA)—drive the rates high enough to make money knowing that the subsidized are immune to huge rate increases but do so at the expense of the 40 % of the market that needs no subsidy. . .
- The cheapest plan available in Florida, a Molina Bronze Obamacare plan, has an annual premium of $13,000 a year for a family of four—mom and dad age 40—with a per person deductible of $8,000. That means that this family would have to incur $21,000 in expenses to qualify for anything other than a preventive care visit." [2]

Such unmitigated joy over how lucrative health care markets are, but with no concern about what all this means to patients and their families!

Surprise medical bills have become a huge concern in the last several years across the country. According to a 2018 tracking poll by the Kaiser Family Foundation, four in ten adults reported that they had a surprise medical bill from a physician, hospital, or laboratory over the past year, with more than one-third very worried that they could not afford to pay them. [3] Figure 8.1 shows that unexpected medical bills are the leading reason for the public to worry, far exceeding such essentials as rent/mortgage, transportation costs, monthly utilities, and food.

FIGURE 8.1

UNEXPECTED MEDICAL BILLS TOP LIST OF PUBLIC'S WORRIES

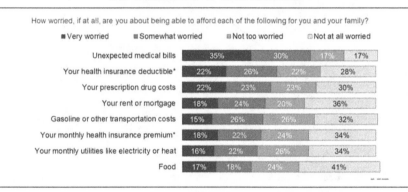

How worried, if at all, are you about being able to afford each of the following for you and your family?

■ Very worried   ■ Somewhat worried   ■ Not too worried   ▢ Not at all worried

	Very worried	Somewhat worried	Not too worried	Not at all worried
Unexpected medical bills	35%	30%	17%	17%
Your health insurance deductible*	22%	26%	22%	28%
Your prescription drug costs	22%	23%	23%	30%
Your rent or mortgage	18%	24%	20%	36%
Gasoline or other transportation costs	15%	26%	26%	32%
Your monthly health insurance premium*	18%	22%	24%	34%
Your monthly utilities like electricity or heat	16%	22%	26%	34%
Food	17%	18%	24%	41%

Source: Kaiser Family Foundation Health Tracking Poll, conducted February 13-18, 2020

There's a battle royal going on now, mostly behind the scenes, by corporate and physician interests lobbying against each other as they try to influence any possible legislation that might emerge from Congress to rein in high surprise medical bills. Insurers are trying to pay less for a fix, hospitals are wanting to protect themselves from cuts, and physician organizations are lobbying to protect their reimbursement, especially the specialty groups most involved in high out-of-network bills. Four medical organizations have been most active—the American College of Emergency Physicians, Envision Care, U. S. Acute Care Solutions, and U. S. Anesthesia Partners—which gave some $1.1 million in 2019 to members of Congress. The battle is further clouded in that these organizations are backed by private equity firms, which are committed to retaining profits from these high bills. [4]

Figure 8.2 gives us an interesting way to see how we compare with the global distribution of population and health spending. Again, we're the leaders in the wrong direction! With just 4 percent of the world's population, we account for 43 percent of health care spending.

FIGURE 8.2

GLOBAL DISTRIBUTION OF POPULATION AND HEALTH SPENDING, 2017

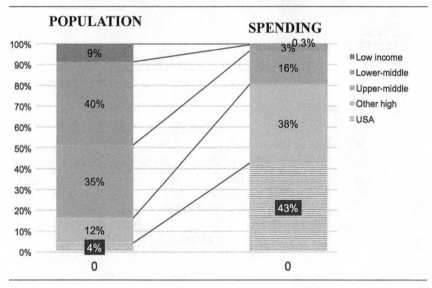

Source: Kutzen, J, and New Perspectives on Global Health Spending for Universal Health Coverage. World Health Organization, 2017.

II. Profiteering, Corruption, and Fraud Across the Medical-Industrial Complex

Let's take a quick tour around many parts of our health care system with a view to how they maximize profits through their business 'ethic,' at times through corruption and even fraud, with little regard for meeting patients' needs for affordable care. Here are some of the ways that each of these parts of our health care system game the system for higher revenues:

1. Hospitals

- Merging into large consolidated hospital systems whereby they gain near monopoly levels and can charge what the traffic will bear [5]
- The most profitable "non-profit" hospitals tend to be part of big, consolidated hospital systems, allowing them to charge more with their large market shares. [6]
- Charging double or even triple what Medicare would pay. [7]
- Up-coding for more billing codes, especially in their affiliated clinics, whether or not care was provided for them; medical billing fraud has been estimated to account for about $270 billion a year. [8]
- Paying high kickbacks to employed physicians in return for them bringing more referrals; paying some as if they are full-time when they work much less, or paying them up to four times what their peers earn; often these practices lead to litigation; [9]
- Not admitting patients and keeping them in observation status, sometimes for days, during which patients face copayments for individual tests and services. [10]
- Repeating a CT scan in an ER for $9000, despite the fact that a similar scan had been done just a few weeks earlier for $268. [11]

2. Ambulance services
- Costs of air ambulance flights have soared since private equity firms began buying up ambulance companies in the wake of the 2008 recession. Two of the three largest air ambulance companies are private equity owned. Investigators have found that about 80 percent of these flights are not emergencies, but lucrative to the owners. [12]

3. Nursing homes
- Discharging or evicting patients when they become sicker and need more care. [13]
- Private equity firms pooling money from investors, borrowing even more, then buying, revamping, and selling off nursing home companies. As we saw on page 35, the Carlyle Group did just that in buying ManorCare, the second biggest nursing home chain in the U. S., then cutting staff, being cited for health code violations and harm to patients, and filing for bankruptcy. [14]

- Overbilling Medicare and the Federal Employees Health Benefits Program for medically unnecessary rehabilitation services, as Guardian Elder Care Holdings did, operating more than 50 nursing facilities in three states, and for which they had to settle with the federal government for more than $15 million to resolve False Claims Act allegations from a whistleblower filing. [15]

4. PhRMA:

- Exorbitant increases in drug prices, such as for Duraprim, often used by patients with HIV, from $13.30 to $750 per tablet in 2016; Martin Shkreli, the CEO of the manufacturer, was later found guilty on two counts of security fraud. [16]
- Big pharmacy chains profiting from the opioid epidemic by ordering huge quantities of prescription opioid pills. (Figure 8.3)
- Making secret deals with drug makers and pharmacy benefit managers, such as CVS Caremark and Express Scripts, that drive higher prices for prescription drugs as they accelerate through corporate mergers. [17]

FIGURE 8.3

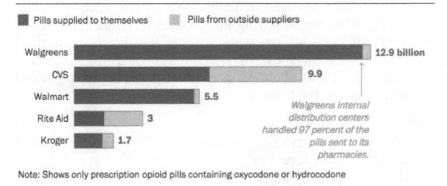

PAIN PILLS ORDERED BY THE TOP FIVE PHARMACY CHAINS

■ Pills supplied to themselves   ■ Pills from outside suppliers

Walgreens — 12.9 billion
CVS — 9.9
Walmart — 5.5
Rite Aid — 3
Kroger — 1.7

Walgreens internal distribution centers handled 97 percent of the pills sent to its pharmacies.

Note: Shows only prescription opioid pills containing oxycodone or hydrocodone

Source: Mayes, B.R, Emamdjomeh, A, *The Washington Post,* November 11, 2019

- Making arrangements between drug makers and patient assistance charities, involving some of the biggest names in PhRMA, that were actually disguised kickbacks to Medicare patients to cover their out-of-pocket costs for the drugs. [18]
- Drug manufacturers avoiding less profitable drugs and vaccines to the point that we have insufficient availability of such essential products as immune globulin and the vaccine for shingles. [19]

5. Physicians' conflicts of interest and collusion with industry and corporate systems

Profiteering physicians, in collusion with industry and corporate interests, work behind the scenes in various ways, as illustrated by the following examples:

- Physician ownership of facilities, such as specialty hospitals, ambulatory surgery centers, and imaging centers, are ways for physician owners to maximize their revenues by charging for services, sharing in a facility profit, and increasing the value of their investment in the business to get around anti-kickback regulations. These conflicts of interest, of course, typically lead to more services being provided than are necessary. It has been found, for example, that physician owners of CT and other imaging centers order two to eight times as many imaging procedures as those who do not own such equipment, amounting to an estimated $40 billion worth of unnecessary imaging each year. [20]
- Physicians accepting payments for patient referrals in violation of the Anti-Kickback Statute. As one example, Boston Heart Diagnostics Corporation recently had to settle with the government for more than $26 million for two whistleblower claims that it generated more income for participating hospitals and itself by coordinating with hospitals' independent marketers to offer physicians money in exchange for referrals. [21]
- Physicians are paid large amounts of money from industry every year for promotional talks and "consulting" that are really disguised marketing strategies. More than 2,500 U. S. physicians have taken in at least $500,000 in the last five years from drug and medical device companies for this purpose, with more than 700 physicians accounting for more than $1 million each. [22]

6. Private health insurers

Health insurers have many ways to profiteer on the backs of their enrollees, in both private plans and privatized Medicare and Medicaid managed care plans. These are some of them:

- Imposing higher co-pays and deductibles, which they rationalize as giving patients "more skin in the game," restricting choice through narrowed networks of physicians and hospitals, limiting expensive drugs on changing drug formularies, and denial of claims, which average 18 percent of claims under the ACA. [23]

- Private Medicare Advantage plans take in revenues that are 30 percent higher than what they spend on care, amounting to about $200 billion a year. [24, 25] For many years, they have gamed the system through high overpayments, partly by paying vendors to find additional billing codes for which claims are made without care being provided. Figure 4.2 on page 45 shows that pattern from 2008 to 2016. Table 8.1 summarizes a pervasive upcoding scam in privatized Medicare Advantage plans.

TABLE 8.1

HMO "HOUSE CALLS"
A NEW UPCODING SCAM

- HMOs send its "housecall" doctor – or one from Mobile Medical Examination Services Inc.

- Doctor seeks out unimportant diagnoses, e.g. mild arthritis

- No treatment offered

- Extra diagnoses allow HMOs to upcode - adding > $3 billion/yr to Medicare Advantage payments

- Efforts to outlaw upcoding "housecalls" were scrapped after industry lobbying blitz

Source: Schulte, Center for Public Integrity, 2014

- Overpayments to private Medicaid managed care plans are endemic in more than 30 states, often involving unnecessary or duplicative payments to providers. [26] These plans often outsource the work of "coordinating" enrollees' care to subcontractors (that may be owned by private equity firms), who make money by denying or skimping on services. [27]
- Making money from the coronavirus pandemic through not covering the costs of treatment, just the costs of testing, which the federal government will compensate them for. [28]

7. Addiction rehabilitation programs

With death rates from drug overdoses more than triple what they were 20 years ago, it is difficult to find an effective and reliable rehabilitation program. These are ways that some so-called rehab centers fraudulently prey on patients:

- Paying "body brokers" thousands of dollars to troll social media and sobriety meetings for insured people who need treatment.
- Plying patients with drugs between times in rehab in order to recycle them back into "treatment." [29]

8. Laboratory tests

As the opioid epidemic continues across the country and without national standards for who gets tested, for what drugs and how often, fraud has become a big problem with many doctor-owned testing clinics charging high billings to Medicare and other payers. One example: Comprehensive Pain Specialists, with a network of 54 such clinics, billed Medicare more than $11 million for urine and related tests in 2014, [30]

Another current example of deceptive marketing, attempted profiteering and even fraud involves direct-to-consumer marketing of "at home" testing kits for Covid-19. The FDA has not authorized any of these tests for at home use. One obvious scam is when consumers are promised an almost immediate test result. [31]

9. Home health

As home health care has become a big industry, fraud has likewise come along with it, taking many forms, such as:

- home health agencies billing for false work
- illegitimate certificates of "training"
- kickbacks to primary care physicians from home health agencies
- falsification of patients' diagnoses as needs for care
- agencies discharging patients and then re-admitting them at the same or related agency without an intervening change in the patient's medical condition. [32, 33]

10. Medical information

This is another huge industry, and these two examples reveal new areas for profiteering and fraud:

- Dozens of whistleblower lawsuits have been filed by physicians and hospitals alleging that EHR software has hidden defects that were concealed during government-mandated reviews intended to ensure safety. As a result, users of the electronic medical record were often unable to track drug prescriptions or doses accurately, thereby putting their patients at risk. Three major EHR vendors ended up paying a total of $357 million in settlements to close the books on allegations that they rigged or otherwise gamed the government's certification tests. [34]
- Quantum Health is a digital provider of medical information and advertising in physicians' offices. It was recently forced to sign a non-prosecution agreement with the Department of Justice to settle allegations that it defrauded its clients (including pharmaceutical companies) by misrepresenting both the quality and quantity of its advertising services. As part of that agreement, it is paying $70 million to victims of its fraud scheme that included its clients, lenders, and investors. [35]

11. Group purchasing organizations (GPOs)

These are organizations, owned by hospitals, that most of us have not heard of that are legally protected from kickback prosecutions under a 1987 law. They sell market share in the form of exclusionary contracts to vendors in return for large kickbacks from suppliers. Phillip Zweig, director of Physicians Against Drug

Shortages, tells us that these GPOs with this safe harbor against kickback prosecutions are fueling the drug shortage crisis and growing prices of generic drugs by extorting big kickbacks from generic drug makers in return for sole source contracts. [36]

12. *"Plassing"*

Here's one more fraud, which crosses international borders, that you may not be aware of. Spain's Barcelona-based Grifols family sells blood plasma in some 220 collection centers in at least 32 states, mostly located in low-income areas. It takes in some $100 million each year, but pays donors only $70 for a pint and a half of plasma. Most donors just need the money. Drugs derived from plasma are then used for treating such conditions as hemophilia. It is legal in this country to pay these donors as the Grifols family has amassed a $3.8 billion fortune. [37]

III. Waste vs. Patient Care

After this exploitive tour through much of our health care "system," we are left to conclude that underlying market forces, fueled by Wall Street investors and private equity firms, keep driving prices and costs higher on the backs of patients, families, and taxpayers. So much of this is waste, and it is unsustainable. But we have to remember that our costs are profits to Wall Street investors, corporate stakeholders, and other middle parties, so that any reform will be hard-fought by deep-pocket interests.

Here are markers that show how seriously ill our health care system has become:

- Up to one-third of health care services provided in the U. S. are inappropriate or unnecessary, with some even harmful. [38]
- Up to one-half of medical procedures provided by physicians each year are not supported by best scientific evidence. [39]
- In contrast to other advanced countries, the U. S. has not adopted any kind of a system for evaluating treatments by cost-effectiveness, largely due to strong political opposition from corporate stakeholders.
- Hospital billing and administrative functions now consume one-third of health care expenditures in the U. S., more than four times the amount spent in Canada with its single-payer financing system. (Figure 8.4) [40]

- Malcolm Sparrow, author of the 2000 classic book, *License to Steal: How Fraud Bleeds America's Health Care System,* whom we met in earlier chapters, estimates that massive billing fraud now consumes at least $350 billion a year. [41]
- Primary care physician practices now have to pay $99,000 per year per physician in their non-clinical administrative activities; physician practices have to devote one staff day per week just to maintain and update provider directories. [42]
- The Centers for Medicare and Medicaid Services (CMS) project that more than $2.7 trillion will be spent by the federal government for private health insurance overhead and administration of government programs (mostly Medicare and Medicaid) between 2014 and 2022, including $273.6 billion in *new administrative costs* for the ACA's expanded Medicaid program. [43]

FIGURE 8.4

HOSPITAL BILLING AND ADMINISTRATION, U.S. AND CANADA, 2019

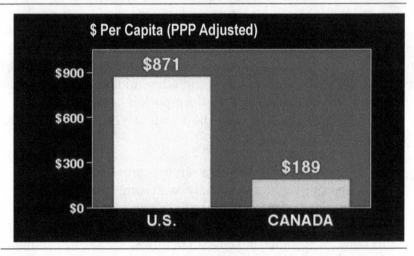

Source: Woolhandler et al *NEJM* 2003; Himmelstein et al, *Health Affairs* 9/2014

Conclusion

After this stark assessment of system challenges in this country, we move to the next chapter, where we will consider the adverse impacts on patients, health care professionals, and taxpayers.

References:

1. Rosenthal, E. Analysis: Choosing a plan from the impossible health care maze. *Kaiser Health News*, December 6, 2019.
2. Laszewski, B. Profitability in the health care marketplace has never been better. *Health Care Policy and Marketplace Review*, February 5, 2020.
3. Kaiser Family Foundation. A polling surprise? Americans rank unexpected medical bills at the top of family budget worries, February 28, 2020. (August 23-28, 2018, Peterson-Kaiser Health System Tracker.
4. Pradhan, R. When your doctor is also a lobbyist: Inside the war over surprise medical bills. *Kaiser Health News*, February 12, 2020.
5. Abelson, R. When hospitals merge to save money, patients often pay more. *New York Times*, November 14, 2018.
6. Ofri, D. Why are nonprofit hospitals so highly profitable? *New York Times*, February 20, 2020.
7. Abelson, R. Many hospitals charge double or even triple what Medicare would pay. *New York Times*, May 9, 2019.
8. Private health care as an act of terrorism. *Common Dreams*, July 20, 2015, p. 1.
9. Rau, J. Hospitals accused of paying doctors large kickbacks in quest for patients. *Kaiser Health News*, May 31, 2019.
10. Graham, J. Even doctors can't navigate our 'broken health care system.' *Kaiser Health News*, May 2, 2019.
11. Rosenthal, E. Year one of KHN's 'Bill of the Month:' A financial kaleidoscope of financial challenges. *Kaiser Health News*, December 21, 2019.
12. Castagno, P. How private equity exploited ambulances and vulnerable patients. *Citizen Truth*, October 3, 2019.
13. Bernard, TS, Pear, R. Complaints about nursing home evictions rise, and regulators take note. *New York Times*, February 22, 2018.
14. Whoriskey, P, Keating, D. Overdoses, bedsores, broken bones: What happened when a private-equity firm sought to care for society's most vulnerable? *The Washington Post,* November 25, 2018.
15. Guardian Elder Care to pay $15.4 million to settle False Claims Act charges. *Corporate Crime Reporter* 34:8, February 24, 2020.
16. Emett, A. A Big PhRMA raises price of cancer drug by 1,400 percent. *Nation of Change*, December 27, 2017.
17. Serafini, M, Barrett, R. Secret deals drive higher prescription drug costs. *Tarbell*, May 24, 2018.
18. Silverman, E. Sanofi to pay nearly $12 million for illegally using a charity to pay kickbacks to Medicare patients. *STAT*, February 28, 2020.
19. Loftus, P. Medicine shortfall hits many patients. *Wall Street Journal*, August 10-11, 2019: A3.
20 Bach, P. Paying doctors to ignore patients. *New York Times*, July 24, 2008.
21. Lab to pay $26.67 million to settle False Claims Act charges. *Corporate Crime Reporter*, December 9, 2019.
22. Ornstein, C, Weber, T, Jones, RG. We found over 700 doctors who were paid more than a million dollars by drug and medical device companies. *ProPublica*, October 17, 2019.
23. Silvers, JB. This is the most realistic path to Medicare for All. *New York*

Times, October 16, 2019.

24. Kronick, R. Why Medicare Advantage plans are being overpaid by $200 billion and what to do about it. *Health Affairs Blog*, January 29, 2020.

25. Curto, V, Einav, L, Finkelstein, A et al. Health care spending and utilization in public and private Medicare. *American Economic Journal: Applied Economics*, April 2019.

26. Herman, B. Medicaid's unmanaged managed care. *Modern Healthcare*, April 30, 2016.

27. Terhune, C. Coverage denied: Medicaid patients suffer as layers of private companies profit. *Kaiser Health News*, January 3, 2019.

28. Potter, W. Coronavirus pandemic reveals just how devastating the greed of for-profit insurance industry has become. *Common Dreams*, March 18, 2020.

29. Wolfson, BJ. Good rehab is hard to find. *Kaiser Health News*, February 5, 2020.

30. Schulte, F, Lucas, E. Liquid gold: Pain doctors soak up profits by screening urine for drugs. *Kaiser Health News*, November 6, 2017.

31. Knight, V. Online coronavirus tests are just the latest iffy products marketed to anxious consumers. *Kaiser Health News*, March 31, 2020.

32. Confessore, N, Kershaw, S. As home health industry booms, little oversight to counter fraud. *New York Times*, September 2, 2007.

33. Lee, SC. Assistant United States Attorney (ND-IL). Law-enforcement observations about home-health fraud, 2020.

34. Schulte, R, Fry, E. Electronic health records creating a 'new era' of health care fraud. *Kaiser Health News*, December 23, 2019.

35. Outcome Health gets non-prosecution agreement to pay $70 million to resolve fraud investigation. *Corporate Crime Reporter*, November 19, 2019, pp. 9-10.

36. Phillip Zweig on Blumenthal Delrahim GPOs and the safe harbor. *Corporate Crime Reporter* 34 (7), February 17, 2020: 1-3.

37. Vickers, E. Family builds $3.8 billion fortune, one pint of blood at a time. *Bloomberg*, February 10, 2020.

38. Gerber, AS, Patashnik, EM, Doherty, D et al. The public wants information, not board mandates, from comparative effectiveness research. *Health Affairs* 29 (10): 1879, 2010.

39. AAMC Government Relations. *Summary of Patient Outcomes Research Provisions*, March 2010.

40. Himmelstein, DU, Campbell, T, Woolhandler, S et al. Landmark administrative waste study updated. Health care administrative costs in the United States and Canada, 2017.

41. Sparrow, M. As quoted by Nader, R. 25 ways the Canadian Health Care System is Better than Obamacare for the 2020 Elections. *Common Dreams*, September 19, 2019.

42. Bannow, T. Physician practices spend one staff day per week on provider directory upkeep. *Modern Healthcare*, November 14, 2019.

43. Himmelstein, DU, Woolhandler, S. The post-launch problem: The Affordable Care Act's persistently high administrative costs. *Health Affairs Blog*, May 27, 2015.

Chapter 9

HARM TO PATIENTS, HEALTH CARE PROFESSIONALS, TAXPAYERS AND THE HEALTH CARE SYSTEM

The excess cost of American healthcare goes to hospitals, to doctors, to device manufacturers, and to drug manufacturers. The trillion dollars that, from a health perspective, is waste and abuse is, from the providers' perspective, well-earned income. Which leaves us with two questions: What effects do these costs have on Americans' lives, and how does the industry manage to get away with it? [1]

—Anne Case, Ph.D. and Angus Deaton, Ph.D., Professors emeritus of Economics and Public Affairs at Princeton University and co-authors of the 2020 book, *Deaths of Despair and the Future of Capitalism*

The above summary of how misdirected the U. S. health care system is from what should be its main purpose—best meeting the needs of patients and their families—is spot on, as are Drs. Case and Deaton's questions. Here we will deal with their first question and will address their second question in the chapter to follow.

This chapter has three goals: (1) to describe the harm to patients in this misdirected, profit-driven system; (2) to consider how physicians and other health professionals have been adversely impacted; and (3) to assess the increasing burdens on taxpayers and harm to the health care system itself.

1. Harm to Patients in our Broken System

To start us off, let's look at two exorbitant medical bills that illustrate not just prevalent medical billing fraud, but also how difficult or impossible it is for those who receive these bills to understand them, much less cope with them.

- Steven Brill, attorney and journalist, had the misfortune of requiring emergency surgery for an aortic aneurism in 2014. He had good insurance through Aetna, the third largest insurer in the country, but his bills for eight days in the hospital came to $197,000. He could not get explanations of his many bills, even after showing them to Aetna's CEO. That motivated him to write the important 2015 book, *America's Bitter Pill: Money, Politics, Backroom Deals, and the Fight to Fix Our Broken Health Care System.* Noting how the ACA had done nothing to rein in health care costs, he described the reasons this way:

  > *It's about money: Healthcare is America's largest industry by far, employing a sixth of the country's workforce. And it is the average American family's largest single expense, whether paid out of their pockets or through taxes and insurance premiums. . . In a country that treasures the marketplace . . . how much taming can we do when the healthcare industry spends four times as much on lobbyists as the number two Beltway spender, the much-feared military-industrial complex.*[2]

- Dr. Elizabeth Rosenthal, whom we met in the last chapter, had the same problem in trying to understand the medical bills for her husband after his bicycle accident. The bill for two days in intensive care was over $9,000, plus many other bills for physicians and others they never met. The biggest single part of his ER bill was a so-called "trauma activation fee" (more than $7,000). That has been allowed since 2002, when the Trauma Association of America, a trade group, successfully lobbied for it as compensation for maintaining a "state of readiness." Dr. Rosenthal categorized these many bills in three ways—*medical swag* (or plunder), the *cover charge, impostor billing*, the *drive-by*, and the *enforced upgrade*. This is how she summed up this situation:

  > *These are all everyday, normal experiences in today's health care system, and they may be perfectly legal. If we want to tame the costs in our $3 trillion health system, we've got to rein in this behavior, which is fraud by any other name.*[3]

Surprise medical bills have reached epidemic proportions in this country, with no fix yet on the horizon—and unlikely until we have system financing reform. (Figure 9.1) The battle for more revenue continues among the main players at the negotiating table—hospitals, physicians, and insurers. Each group keeps adding up its own way to gain further income—such as facility fees for hospitals, increased cost-sharing and narrowed networks for insurers, and physicians walking away from networks in order to charge what they want out-of-network.

FIGURE 9.1

ONE IN FIVE INSURED ADULTS HAD A SURPRISE MEDICAL BILL IN THE PAST TWO YEARS

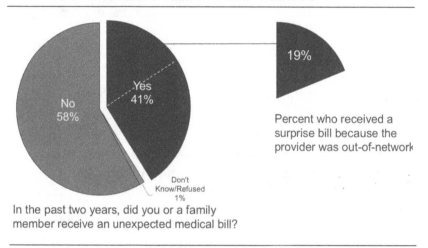

19%

Percent who received a surprise bill because the provider was out-of-network

Yes 41%

No 58%

Don't Know/Refused 1%

In the past two years, did you or a family member receive an unexpected medical bill?

Source: Kaiser Family Foundation, and *The Journal of the American Medical Association*

All of this ends up hurting patients as they struggle to deal with their own health care. Here are some of the various ways that they lose along the way, as we've already seen in earlier chapters, including the family straight jacket of medical care costs through the Milliman Medical Index (MMI) (page 54):

• Those with employer sponsored insurance lose wages as their employers cope with rising health care costs; they lose their insurance when they change jobs, and may not regain coverage with another employer.

- Even when one has other private health insurance, it is typically far short of covering one's bills, in which case persons are often forced to delay care and incur worse outcomes later.
- The circumstances become more urgent for the 30 million uninsured and the 87 million *underinsured* Americans.
- Loss of continuity of care due to shortage of primary care physicians and being shuffled about among many physicians who don't know your story.
- Increased inequality and deaths of despair, with decreasing life expectancy among Americans ages 25 to 64. (Figure 9.2)[4]
- Financial hardship, with increasing debt ($88 billion in 2018) (Figure 9.3) [5]
- Crowdfunding, sought by 8 million for family members and another 12 million for non-family members, in order to pay medical bills. [6]
- Private debt collectors, affecting one in three Americans. [7]
- Lawsuits when can't pay [8]
- Medical bankruptcy, accounting for two-thirds of personal bankruptcies, involving 530,000 families each year. [9]

FIGURE 9.2

RISING DEATH RATES IN U.S., AGES 25-64, 2010-2017

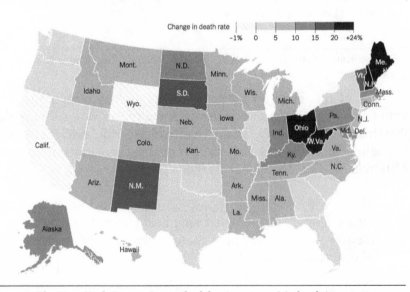

Source: *The New York Times*: *Journal of the American Medical Association*

FIGURE 9.3

HEALTH COSTS FORCE MILLIONS INTO DEBT AND TO FOREGO OTHER ESSENTIALS

Percent of Adults Who Have Borrowed Money or Reduced Spending Due to Health Care Costs

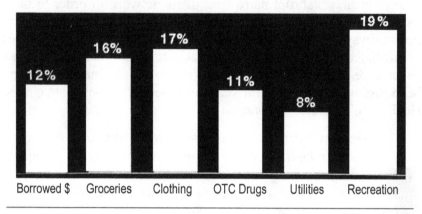

Source: Westhealth/Gallup, Public Perceptions of the Health Care System, 2019

II. Harm to Physicians and Other Health Professionals

Here we will consider some of the main consequences of these trends for physicians, which often further involve nurses and other health professionals as organizational structures change in a consolidating corporate-dominated marketplace.

Although physicians played a dominant role in shaping the directions and content of health care up through the 1960s, they have lost much of their influence over the now dominant corporate based system that has evolved since then. Most physicians today are employed by others, especially by large hospital systems, unlike earlier generations when independent practice prevailed.

As hospital systems acquire physician groups, they of course increase their prices and revenues. The AMA has found that about 60 percent of internists and pediatricians are now employed by hospitals, together with 50 percent of surgeons and 25 percent of surgical subspecialists.[10]

These are some of the adverse impacts of current trends for physicians and other health professionals today.

1. Loss of a long-established medical practice

This physician's experience, as head of a long-standing group practice, illustrates a typical and common change associated with a large insurer's abrupt narrowing of its network in order to have its new network physicians more compliant with its reimbursement rates (always in the insurer's best interests, not those of enrollees or affiliated physicians!). Going back to one of his physician's experience, discussed in Chapter 4 (page 46), Dr. Inas Wassef had been Rasha's pediatrician for years until being dropped from United Healthcare's Medicaid managed care network in 2019.

> *Dr. Alexander Salerno, an internist, has operated his own 17-physician multi-specialty group practice in East Orange, New Jersey, for many years. His main office is in a three-story, 19th century house where his father had conducted his own medical practice in the 1960s. Forty percent of Dr. Salerno's patients are on Medicaid.*
>
> *UnitedHealthcare, one of the largest insurers in the country, has seen a ten-fold increase in its profits and stock prices since 2010, largely through privatized Medicare and Medicaid managed care contracts. Dr. Salerno was initially pleased with the extra benefits under Medicare Advantage that include vision and dental care.*
>
> *Then the plot thickened. Riverside Medical Group, a 20-office physicians' practice in the surrounding area, is owned by Optum, a sister company of United Healthcare, both of which are owned by UnitedHealth Group. When Riverside Medical Group offered to buy the Salerno group practice in 2018, Dr. Salerno declined. UnitedHealthcare gave the Salerno group a $130,000 bonus for its good care of patients in 2019. The next shoe to drop, soon thereafter, was the insurer's abrupt exclusion of his group practice from its network in 2020, leaving many patients in limbo.*
>
> *This situation is now being litigated. The State Department of Human Services has blocked UnitedHealthcare from enrolling any new members to the more than 400,000 members it already has in its Medicaid managed care plan,*

the second-largest in the state. As Dr. Salerno reflects: "It's not a bad insurance company. It just seems like they have become greedy trying to control both ends of the pendulum—wanting to be the payer and the provider." [11]

2. Loss of clinical autonomy

Physician judgments of necessary, even emergency care are often questioned by insurance plan managers, or their clerks. Primary care physicians are especially hard hit by the bureaucracy they have to deal with every day. Before their patients can be seen and treated for a primary care visit, they and their staff have to: (a) verify their patients' insurance, (b) get pre-authorization for planned tests and procedures, (c) find out what drugs are covered by differing formularies among insurers, and (d) determine whether other specialist consultants are in- or out-of -network. Figure 9.4 shows that physicians now spend twice as much time each day on the EHR and deskwork as with patients.

FIGURE 9.4

DOCTORS SPEND TWICE AS MUCH TIME ON EHR/DESK WORK AS WITH PATIENTS

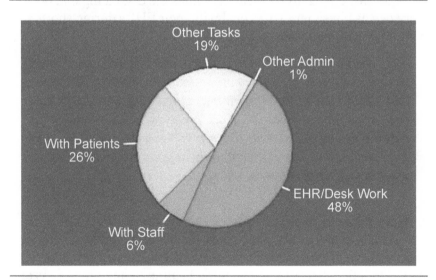

Source: Sinsky et al. *Ann Int Med* 9/20/16

A 2017 survey by the AMA of its members found that 84 percent of respondents found that pre-authorizations were a high or extremely high burden (requiring more than 14 hours a week of staff time), with 92 percent believing that they had a negative impact on patient outcomes. [12] Dr. Halee Fischer-Wright, President and CEO of the Medical Group Management Association, concluded:

> *Health plan demands for approval for physician-ordered medical tests, clinical procedures, medications, and medical devices ceaselessly question the judgment of physicians, resulting in less time to treat patients and needlessly driving up administrative costs for medical groups.* [13]

3. Erosion of physician-patient relationship

Under the pressure from their employers, usually corporate hospital systems, physicians are pressured to upcode for maximal revenue, deal with the increased bureaucracy of insurers, and see more patients in less time. All that has led to limited face-to-face and listening time with patients as their physicians have to also deal with electronic health records on their computers. By 1997, primary care physicians were spending an average of just 8 minutes talking to a patient during an office visit, less than one-half the time spent ten years earlier. [14] This incident illustrates the distancing that occurs every day as physicians try to deal with their EHRs during shortened visit times with patients.

> *The family physician of a friend, age 88, was out of town, so in his absence she saw another doctor whom she had never met. After a ten-minute appointment, he stood up to leave, and she asked him: "What color are my eyes?" Taken aback, he asked why she asked that. Her reply: "You did not look at me once during our appointment, only at your computer. I never want another appointment with you."*

4. Moral harm to physicians.

With a majority of physicians increasingly beholden to and employed by revenue-driven systems of care that give them less time to practice their time-consuming healing, many physicians are experiencing moral injury from the pervasive values of the system around them. Dr. Kenneth Ludmerer, internist, medical historian and Professor of Medicine at Washington University in St. Louis, called attention to this problem in his 1999 book, *Time to Heal: American Medical Education from the Turn of the Century to the Era of Managed Care* in these words:

> *Perhaps the most extraordinary development in medical practice during the age of managed care was that time, in the name of efficiency, was being squeezed out of the doctor-patient relationship. Managed care organization, with their insistence on maximizing "throughput," were forcing physicians to churn through patients in assembly-line fashion at ever-accelerating speeds . . many doctors were staggering under the load.* [15]

5. Increasing burnout and suicides

Predictably, these pressures have contributed to dissatisfaction, burnout, and impaired mental health of physicians. A national study by Medscape, its 2019 National Physician Burnout, Depression and Suicide Report, documented the severe impacts of today's medical practice on U. S. physicians. It found that 44 percent of physicians are burned out, with job stress that leads to exhaustion, feeling overwhelmed, and lacking a sense of personal accomplishment. Their leading reason for this stress was reported as too many bureaucratic tasks, such as charting and paperwork. One in ten were colloquially depressed, with 4 percent clinically depressed. [15]

Physician suicide is not a new problem in the U. S. A 2003 report estimated that 300 physicians were taking their own lives each year. [16] A 2015 study found that 28 percent of medical residents had a major depressive episode during their training, almost four times the rate of similarly aged individuals in the U. S. general population.[17] Although depression and suicidality are very treatable, there is a pervasive stigma against mental illness throughout the medical community, and many physicians so affected do not receive care.[18, 19]

6. Early retirement

In reaction to these problems, many more physicians are retiring early. Dr. Valerie Jones, now a retired obstetrician-gynecologist, sums up her reasons for retiring this way, which are likely shared by so many other early retirees:

> *The reach of insurance companies and health care administrators (who are not clinicians) has stealthily worked its way throughout the health care system in the United States and is strangling the lifeblood of physicians. The joy of medicine is being sucked out slowly by increased burdens of pressure to see more, do more, without regard to patient outcome—of course with the caveat of earning more money for the bottom line of the organization, not to the benefit of the patient or physician. . . . The problem occurs when health care becomes a business run by people who are not clinicians. Physicians begin to feel like they are running up against a brick wall. A wall of denials for patient care, refusals of requests for adequate visit time with patients, and a blocking of advocacy for patients by the professionals who can help them most.* [20]

III. Adverse Impacts on Taxpayers and the Health Care System

With all the money sloshing around in the U. S. health care system through profiteering, corruption and fraud, we have to ask where all this money is going? A report from the Institute of Medicine in 2013 answered this question, as of 2009, totaling $765 billion a year, which included: [21]

1. Unnecessary services	$210 billion
2. Inefficiently delivered care	$130 billion
3. Excess administrative costs	$190 billion
4. Excessively high prices	$105 billion
5. Missed prevention opportunities	$55 billion
6. Fraud	$75 billion

We can expect those dollars to be significantly higher today.

Many of us don't realize that we, as taxpayers, fund almost two-thirds of overall U. S. spending on health care. (Figure 9.5)

FIGURE 9.5

TAXES FUND 2/3 OF HEALTH SPENDING

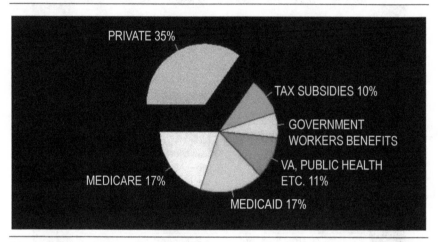

Source: Himmelstein & Woolhandler - Analysis of NCHS data

To gain further insight of what this means, we have to ask a second question—who really pays for health care? Dr. Uwe Reinhardt, well-known economist whom we met in Chapter 5, makes the case that all spending on health care originates from private households. The government accounts for more than 60 percent of health care spending through both public and private plans, but gets the needed funds through taxing household budgets. Private households pay premiums into public or private insurance pools while private employers recoup insurance coverage for their employees by taking money from their household budgets in the form of wage cuts and/or reduction of other fringe benefits. Figure 9.6 shows how money circulates through the system from private households to final payments to providers of care. [22]

Today's system for paying for health care really is rigged against most of the working population as what economists call "labor income," (what Americans earn in their everyday jobs), is taxed even higher than "capital income," (accumulated wealth), which used to be taxed much higher than labor income. [23]

FIGURE 9.6

WHO PAYS FOR HEALTH CARE, AND HOW IS IT PAID?

Ultimately, private households pay for all health care.

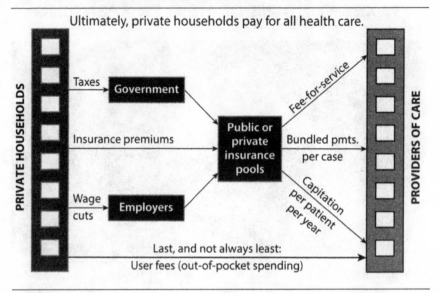

Source: Reinhardt, UE. *Priced Out: The Economic and Ethical Costs of American Health Care*. Princeton, NJ. *Princeton University Press*, 2019, p. 63.

University of California Berkeley economists Emmanuel Saez and Gabriel Zucman trace growing tax injustice over the last century in their excellent 2019 book, *The Triumph of Injustice: How the Rich Dodge Taxes and How to Make Them Pay.* For the first time since 1915, billionaires pay lower tax rates than their secretaries, steel workers, school teachers, and retirees (about 23 percent of their income vs. 50 percent in 1970). Corporate profits are taxed at just 21 percent since the 2018 tax "reform" act. [24]

What do we get for all this money that most of our population pays for health care in this upside down system? As previously described—not much, and way short of enough. For the huge outlays on health care that are breaking family budgets, we get soaring prices and costs, restricted access to care, poor quality and value, worse outcomes with unaffordable care, and unaccountable bureaucracy and waste.

The pervasive drive by corporate stakeholders for maximal revenue throughout our health care system, with less regard for serving patients' real needs, is the Achilles heel of our medical-industrial complex that is rife with profiteering, corruption, and more fraud than most of us recognize. Health care has become a commodity in a largely for-profit marketplace where competition doesn't really work. Physicians and other health care professionals are held hostage by big corporate interests, in concert with Wall Street traders and investors, who have stolen U. S. health care through their "rent-seeking" behavior.

Drs. Case and Deaton, who opened this chapter, further observe:

> *The vast sums that are being spent on health care are an unsustainable drag on the economy, pushing down wages, reducing the number of good jobs, and undermining financing for education, infrastructure, and the provision of public goods and services that are (or might be) provided by federal and state governments. Working-class life is certainly under threat from automation and from globalization, but healthcare costs are both precipitating and accelerating the decline.* [25]

Conclusion

These adverse consequences of unchanging directions in U. S. health care are unsustainable for patients, health care professionals, taxpayers, and the public. Increasing inequality and inequities punish much of our population to benefit corporate stakeholders and the wealthy.

Recouping rampant waste, together with urgently needed financing reform, can rebuild our health care system for the common good. It is achievable, but only if we develop the political will and a larger role of government oriented to public, not private interests. In the next two and final chapters, we will discuss ways, means, and odds of accomplishing that goal.

References:
1. Case, A, Deaton, A. *Deaths of Despair and the Future of Capitalism.* Princeton, NJ. *Princeton University Press*, 2020, p. 202.
2. Brill, S. *America's Bitter Pill: Money, Politics, Backroom Deals, and the Fight to Fix Our Broken Health Care System.* New York. *Random House,* 2015, pp. 7-8.
3. Rosenthal, E. Where the frauds are all legal. *New York Times,* December 7, 2019.
4. Kolata, G, Tavernise, S. It's not just poor white people driving a decline in life expectancy. *The New York Times,* November 26, 2019.

5. Higgins, E. Making money off dysfunction: Bolstering Medicare for All case, survey shows Americans accrued $88 billion in healthcare debt in 2018. *Common Dreams*, April 2, 2019.

6. Cerullo, M. As medical bills soar, more Americans turn to crowdfunding. *CBS News*, February 21, 2020.

7. Turner, J. *A Pound of Flesh: The Criminalization of Private Debt.* American Civil Liberties Union Report, February 21, 2018.

8. Bell, L. The hospital treated these patients. Then it sued them. *New York Times*, September 3, 2019.

9. Himmelstein, DU, Lawless, RM, Thorne, D et al. Medical bankruptcy: Still common despite the Affordable Care Act. *Am J Public Health*, March 2019.

10. Rosenthal, E. Apprehensive, many doctors shift to jobs with salaries. *New York Times*, February 13, 2014.

11. Galewitz, P. Needy patients 'caught in the middle' as insurance titan drops doctors. *Kaiser Health News*, February 25, 2020.

12. AMA. 2017 AMA Prior Authorization Physician Survey, December 2017.

13. Fischer-Wright, H. MGMA. Payer prior authorization requirements on physicians continue rapid escalation: increasing practice overhead and delaying patient care. Poll, May 16, 2017.

14. Goldberg, RM. What's happened to the healing process? *Wall Street Journal*, June 18, 1997: A 22.

15. Kane, L. *Medscape National Physician Burnout, Depression and Suicide Report,* 2019, January 16, 2019.

16. Center, C, Davis, M, Detre, T et al. Confronting depression and suicide in physicians. *JAMA* 289 (23): 3161, 2003.

17. Mata, DA, Ramos, MA, Bansal, N et al. Prevalence of depression and depressive symptoms among resident physicians. *JAMA* 314 (22): 2373, 2015.

18. Brooks, E. Preventing physician distress and suicide. *American Medical Association*, 2018.

19. Gold, K, Sen, A, Schwenk, T. Details on suicide among U. S. physicians: Data from the National Violent Death Reporting System. Gen Hosp Psychiatry 35 (1): 45-49, 2013.

20. Jones, VA. The reasons so many physicians are retiring early. *MEDPAGE TODAY'S Kevin MD.com*, March 6, 2019.

21. *Best Case at Lower Cost.* Washington, D.C. *Institute of Medicine*, 2013, Table 3.1.

22. Reinhardt, UE. *Priced Out: The Economic and Ethical Costs of American Health Care.* Princeton, NJ. *Princeton University Press*, 2019, p. 63.

23. Saez, E, Zucman, G. *The Triumph of Injustice: How the Rich Dodge Taxes and How to Make Them Pay.* New York. *W. W. Norton & Company, Inc.* 2019, p. 93.

24. Ibid #23, p. xi.

25. Ibid # 1, p. 187.

PART IV

CAN THESE ADVERSE IMPACTS BE REVERSED, AND IF SO, HOW?

Some of us decided that the purpose and the reason for government should be the improvement of life for all of its people.

—Francis Perkins, Cabinet member of Franklin D. Roosevelt's administration and driving force behind Social Security, the 40-hour work week, the eight-hour day, minimum wage and unemployment compensation.

The impact of any pandemic goes well beyond lives lost and commerce curtailed. Today, America faces a fundamental choice between defending the status quo and embracing progressive change. The current crisis could prompt redistributive reforms akin to those triggered by the Great Depression and World War II, unless entrenched interests prove too powerful to overcome.

—Walter Scheidel, Professor of Classics and History at Stanford University and author of *The Great Leveler: Violence and the History of Inequality from the Stone Age to the Twenty-First Century.*[1]

Beyond defeating the disease, the great test all countries will soon face is whether current feelings of common purpose will shape society after the crisis. As western leaders learnt in the Great Depression, and after the second world war, to demand collective sacrifice you must offer a social contract that benefits everyone.

Radical reforms—reversing the prevailing policy direction of the last four decades—will need to be put on the table. Governments will have to accept a more active role in the economy. They must see public services as investments rather than liabilities, and look for ways to make labour markets less insecure. Redistribution will again be on the agenda; the privileges of the elderly and wealthy in question. Policies until recently considered eccentric, such as basic income and wealth taxes, will have to be in the mix.

—Editorial Board of *Financial Times* [2]

1. Scheidel, W. Why the wealthy fear pandemics. *New York Times*, April 9, 2020.
2. Editorial Board. *Financial Times*. Virus lays bare the frailty of the social contract. Radical reforms are required to forge a society that will work for all. *New York Times*, April 3, 2020.

Chapter 10

HOW REGULATION OF HEALTH CARE KEEPS FAILING

Health care fraud has not been brought under control because the health care industry has underestimated the complexity of the fraud-control business and has never developed reasonable defenses against fraud. The defenses currently in place may protect against incorrect billing and certain forms of overutilization, but they offer little protection against criminal fraud. Insurers have no way of knowing how much they lose to fraud and have little incentive to find out. Unable to see the magnitude of the problem, public and private programs massively underinvest in control resources. Insurers rely upon fraud-detection and referral mechanisms that barely work. The majority of them lack a coordinated fraud-control strategy, or the organizational infrastructure to carry it out. . . .

The government has so far not found the courage to measure the fraud rate in its major programs. The health care industry's provider associations and lobbyists have worked hard to contain and soften the government's fledgling enforcement campaign; they no doubt fear the possibility of a serious and sustained examination of the broader business practices that pervade the industry. [1]

Malcolm Sparrow drew the above conclusion in 2000 in his landmark book, *License to Steal: How Fraud Bleeds America's Health Care System.* Because of the severe impacts on health care from profiteering, corruption and fraud that we have seen in earlier chapters, it is more than timely to assess whether we have made any progress in the last 20 years.

This chapter has three goals: (1) to bring some historical perspective to this problem; (2) to give some blatant examples of what is happening now under Trump's deregulation policies; and (3) to describe the continuing forces against regulating health care industries.

I. Historical Perspective

As we know, corporatization and growth of for-profit health care have been increasing since the 1970s. Corporate hospital chains were established within a few years after the passage of Medicare and Medicaid in 1965. Wall Street soon took notice and became enamored with the profits to be made as investor-owned facilities and services grew rapidly. Their corporate profits after taxes soared by more than 100-fold between 1965 and 1990. Robert Kuttner, co-founder of *The American Prospect* and author of the important 1999 book, *Everything for Sale: The Virtues and Limits of Markets*, sounded this early alarm:

> *In America, the over-reliance on market logic and market institutions is ruining the health care system. Market enthusiasts fail to tabulate all the costs of relying on market forces to allocate health care—the fragmentation, opportunism, asset rearranging, overhead, under-investment in public health, and the assault on norms of service and altruism. They assume either a degree of self-regulation that the health markets cannot generate, or far-sighted public supervision that contradicts the rest of their world view . . . There is no realm of our mixed economy where markets yield more perverse results.* [2]

General Electric, already a giant player among America's industrial corporations, had sponsored Ronald Reagan's TV career and launched him on the lecture circuit as a crusader against big government. As a sponsor of the right-wing McLaughlin Group and a leading member of the Business Roundtable, GE was (and is!) a major political force nationally with its own lobbying presence within the Beltway. In his 1992 book, *Who Will Tell the People: The Betrayal of American Democracy*, William Greider told us just how big that presence was:

> *General Electric is a conglomerate that, in addition to its productive, profit-making activities, also functions as a ubiquitous political organization. With great sophistication and tenacity, GE represents its own interests in the political arena, as one would expect. But that is not what makes it so influential.*

General Electric also tries to act like a mediating institution—speaking on behalf of others. GE, like many other companies, assumes the burden of representing various groups of other citizens in politics—workers, consumers, shareholders, even other businesses and the well-being of Americans at large. GE has the resources to develop and promote new political ideas and to organize public opinion around its political agenda. It has the capacity to advise and intervene and sometimes veto. It has the power to punish political opponents. It also has the sophistication to lend its good name to worthy causes, such as the Urban League, only remotely related to the company's profits. [3]

Fifteen years after Robert Kuttner's warning in 1999, he summed up how unfavorable the political landscape has been for regulation and health care reform over the last 35 years:

The era since 1981 has been one of turning away from public remediation, toward tax cuts, limited social spending, deregulation, and privatization. None of this worked well, except for the very top. For everyone else, the shift to conservative policies generated more economic insecurity. [4]

Taking another huge corporate player, the pharmaceutical industry, and fast forwarding to the Affordable Care Act after its enactment in 2010, what can we learn about how well industry has been regulated since then? These three examples answer that question, again in the wrong direction:

- Big PhRMA had contributed more than $7.6 billion to the FDA in user fees between 1993 and 2017 (Figure 10.1) [5], and not surprisingly, was getting rapid approvals for new drugs, without having to provide evidence of added efficacy or safety over comparison drugs. These approvals were given despite the fact that almost one-third of drugs approved by the FDA between 2000 and 2010 had to be withdrawn from the market due to safety concerns and risk to the public. [6] The fox is still in the hen house!

- The 21st Century Cures Act was passed by Congress in late 2016 that drastically lowered even more the FDA's standards for approval of new drugs. The previous gold standard for effectiveness of new drugs depended on rigorous random-controlled trials. It was replaced by a new "standard" for "real world evidence," which can be easily gamed by uncontrolled observational data. [7]
- A 2017 report from Public Citizen, *Twenty-Seven Years of Pharmaceutical Industry Criminal and Civil Penalties: 1991 through 2017*, found a steep drop in federal criminal penalties over the past four years for such crimes as drug pricing fraud against state Medicaid programs, unlawfully promoting prescription drugs, concealing the results of company-sponsored studies and/or falsifying data submitted to the federal government, and selling products that failed to meet FDA standards. The worst offenders were GlaxoSmithKline and Pfizer, which paid financial penalties over those years of $7.0 and $4.7 billion, respectively. [8]

FIGURE 10.1

PDUFA USER FEE INCREASE PER FISCAL YEAR

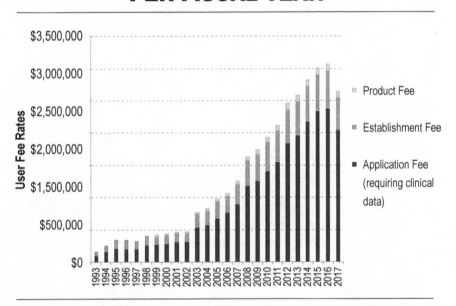

Sources: Avalere Analysis of Prescription Drug User Fee Rates. 1993 - 2017

II. Trump's Deregulation: Misguided Actions or Irresponsible Inaction

A continuing mantra during Trump's presidential campaign and his first three-plus years in office has been to falsely claim that deregulation of health, safety, labor, financial, and environmental sectors will somehow get us on a better track in this country. He issued an executive order just 10 days after his inauguration that government agencies should kill two rules for every one they propose. His Cabinet was then carefully selected for those loyal to "deconstruction of the administrative state," with the strong support of the Freedom Caucus, many trade organizations, and corporate lobbyists. [9]

Ineffective as regulation was in earlier years, it is even more so now under Trump. Here are examples which show how industry-friendly his administration is.

1. FDA drug approvals

At a White House briefing in late March 2020, with the coronavirus pandemic in a rapid climb in cases (more than 50,000 in the U. S.), Trump touted the use of hydroxichloroquine, an anti-malarial drug, for the treatment of COVID-19. It had not been approved by either the FDA in this country or recommended by the World Health Organization. [10] Soon after Trump's reckless announcement encouraging the use of chloroquine as a possible 'game changer' for the prevention or treatment of COVID-19, a couple in Arizona ingested a form of the drug, hydroxychloroquine phosphate. He died of a cardiac arrest within 30 minutes and she was hospitalized in critical condition. [11]

This is a good example of how important scientific evidence is for taking any drug. The rapid emergency approval later by the FDA cited no supporting evidence, no rigorous drug trials had reported results, and experts warn of the dangers of the drug, especially for cardiac arrest. Alex Azar, Trump's appointee as head of DHHS, headed Eli Lilly's U. S. Division from 2012 to 2017, during which he presided over a more than double price increase for its insulin drug. He praised Trump for his "bold leadership," which soon led to Novartis and Bayer contributing millions of doses of this drug to the Strategic National Stockpile. [12]

At about the same time, the FDA granted orphan drug status to Gilead Sciences, manufacturer of remdesivir, an intravenous anti-viral drug, although its efficacy and safety for treating COVID-19 are still unknown. That approval was limited, however, for about 250 seriously ill coronavirus patients under an emergency provision of the agency's "compassionate use" program, which permits the use of new, unapproved drugs without clinical trials when no other treatments are available. That decision gave Gilead tax breaks, waiver of FDA fees, and market exclusivity for seven years. [13]

Beyond there being no documented efficacy or safety for this drug in patients with coronavirus, the orphan drug approval is not intended to be used when its target population is more than 200,000 people (almost certainly the case with COVID-19) and without regulation of its cost for large populations. This is the same Gilead that lobbied successfully to get more rapid approval of Sovaldi for the treatment of Hepatitis C, then pricing it at $84,000 for a full course of treatment! [14] The concern about future profiteering on remdesivir by Gilead is increased by this statement by Alex Azar: "We can't control that price because we need the private sector to invest." [15]

Fortunately, after an immediate backlash from Public Citizen and 50 groups demanding that Gilead relinquish its government-sanctioned monopoly guarantee for a potential COVID-19 treatment, it backed down. Public Citizen's scathing statement cut to the core of our market-based "system":

> *Calling COVID-19 a rare disease mocks people's suffering and exploits a loophole in the law to profiteer off a deadly pandemic. Making the claim to special orphan status even more outrageous is the fact that the public already has largely paid for remdesivir's development through at least $60 million in grants and innumerable contributions from federal scientists. America, and the world, has the right to expect better from Gilead.* [16]

2. Nursing homes, relaxed oversight

The current deadly circumstances of the coronavirus pandemic bring more urgency to re-visiting the matter of regulation. The Centers for Medicare and Medicaid (CMS), even weeks into this disaster, is still undecided after a year's consideration about a proposed rule change, heavily lobbied for by industry, that would relax protections against infections in the nation's nursing homes.

As is now well-known, the Life Care Center of America's nursing home in Kirkland, Washington was the epicenter of the initial outbreak, with a total lack of infection protections that took the lives of 27 out of its 120 residents. [17] When asked recently about the status of a rule that would eliminate a national requirement to have even a part-time infection prevention specialist on each nursing home's staff, Seema Verma, CMS Administrator, could still only say that "the proposed rule change is not about easing up on nursing homes but about not micromanaging the process, and we have to make sure that we get it right for the sake of patients." [18]

3. Delay to invoke the Defense Production Act to meet emergency needs to fight coronavirus pandemic

After downplaying the threat of the coronavirus threat for far too long, Trump finally declared that we are going to war against it. The numbers of confirmed cases and deaths continued to soar, with states pleading with the federal government to address the dire shortage of ventilators, gowns, protective masks and other critical needs. After previously considering invoking the 1950 Defense Production Act to rapidly increase production and distribute them to areas most in need, he changed his mind.[19] Instead, he would depend on the private sector to deal with the problem.

As a result, pressure was building for action due to continued severe shortages, preventable deaths of patients and health care workers, and states bidding against each other. [20] He finally did invoke the Defense Production Act, but in a bizarre and unclear way described by an article in *Daily Kos*—ordering General Motors to make ventilators rapidly, without a contract, with the numbers and prices unstated, and at a factory that GM closed and sold the previous year! [21]

Figure 10.2 illustrates Trump's inability to take responsibility for his Administration's incompetence, indecision, and failure to use the power of his office to deal with this national emergency.

FIGURE 10.2

SHIFTING BLAME FOR COVID-19

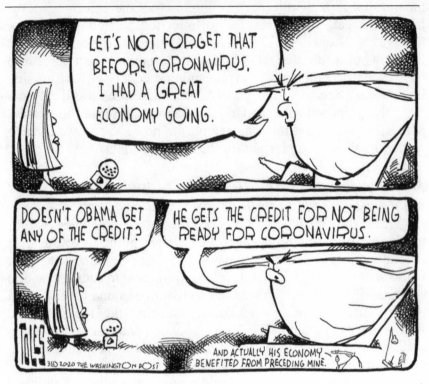

Source: Tom Toles/*The Washington Post*

4. Corporate crime and misconduct

According to a Violation Tracker tool developed by Good Jobs First to track corporate crime and misconduct, federal penalties imposed on America's largest corporations plunged during Trump's first 12 months in office. As part of his deregulatory bonanza, Trump's $1.5 trillion tax cut in 2017 brought them even more profits. [22] Corporate repeat offenders are also given a pass through deferred and non-prosecution agreements, with less enforcement under Trump's Department of Justice. [23]

5. Tax policy

Breaking with long tradition, Trump has been the first presidential candidate not to release his tax returns. When asked by Hillary Clinton during their 2016 presidential campaigns about not paying any tax when he was trying to get a casino license, he replied: "That makes me smart." That attitude harkens back to Ronald Reagan, who compared our tax code to "daily mugging." [24] No wonder, then, that Trump's 2017 tax cut favored corporations and their shareholders more than the rest of us.

III. Forces Aligned Against Regulation

The debate in Congress over stimulus/relief packages once again brought payouts to the wealthy front and center for corporate America versus the interests and needs of middle and lower-income people. We saw a huge increase in corporate lobbying on several fronts, drawing some sectors of the medical-industrial complex together. One little-noticed provision of the sausage bill that emerged was an *accelerated* FDA review of over-the-counter drugs and sunscreen products, as lobbied for by the Public Access to SunScreens Coalition, which has been a priority for Senate Majority Leader McConnell from Kentucky, where cosmetics company L'Oreal has a factory. [25]

These four examples illustrate what's happening on the frontlines of the ongoing battle between corporate stakeholders, government and the public interest.

1. Medical billing reform

According to a 2018 tracking poll by the Kaiser Family Foundation, four in ten adults say that they had a surprise bill from a physician, hospital or laboratory in the past year. Almost 40 percent of patients say they are "very worried" when they receive them. [26] Sirens are blowing for opposing forces as proposals to regulate these surprise bills move through Congress and state legislatures with rare bipartisan support.

New coalitions are forming up to oppose regulatory action. Hospitals are active defenders of surprise bills, which often involve large bills from out-of-network physicians, since they contract with private physician staffing firms to staff emergency rooms and operate physician practices. Because these staffing firms are often private equity firms with ties to venture capital, well funded lobbyists join the fight in an effort to tamp down this hot issue during the 2020 election cycle. [27]

At the beginning of 2020, multiple committees in Congress were working on the problem of how out-of-network payments might be settled between hospitals, insurers and physicians. Two possible approaches have been under consideration—arbitration through independent review to determine a fair price, and benchmarking, whereby physicians would be paid based on an average of what other in-network physicians in the area are paid. As expected, many coalitions are now active in opposing both approaches. The opposition includes hospitals, insurers, physician groups in various specialties, and employers, with the support of large amounts of money from Wall Street. [28] Don't hold your breath about the outcome of this battle, and expect it to be on the side of money, not patients.

2. Hospital pricing

Another hot battle is being waged among hospitals in response to a proposed rule by the Trump administration that would require hospitals to disclose the secret rates negotiated with insurers for all services, including supplies and care provided by physicians who work for their facilities. [29] In response, the American Hospital Association and other industry groups filed a lawsuit in U. S. District Court in Washington, D.C., citing that this rule would violate their First Amendment rights and go beyond the statutory intent of the ACA. [30]

3. Drug pricing

With the prices of prescription drugs at an all-time high and increasingly unaffordable for Americans, even for those with insurance, the drug industry finds itself backed into a corner against growing opposition. Lowering drug prices has become one of the rare reasons uniting Democrats and Republicans. By July of 2019, political action committees run by employees of drug companies and their trade groups had given, in the preceding six months, almost $845,000 to 30 senators expected to run for re-election in 2020. PhRMA's pitch was to support candidates from both political parties who "support innovation and patient access to medicines." [31] PhRMA has also made increasing use of Facebook ads, reaching almost a billion dollars in 2019, and raising concerns about privacy of personal health records. [32]

Big PhRMA has long claimed that their prices are needed to cover the cost of research and development of new drugs and vaccines. But this claim is specious for two reasons—they greatly exaggerate their R &D costs (much of which is not rigorous research) and the National Institutes of Health bear most of the costs. Drug companies avoid less lucrative public health needs, such as vitally needed vaccines.

As Zain Rizvi, law and policy researcher in Public Citizen's Access to Medicines program, recently said:

> *The coronavirus outbreak should be a wake-up call. We cannot depend on monopolies to deliver the medicines we need.* [33]

4. Fighting against Medicare for All

As universal coverage under Medicare for All is taking center stage in the 2020 election cycle, with two bills in Congress (S. 1804 in the Senate and H. R. 1384 in the House), the Trump administration, GOP and corporate stakeholders joined forces to fight against it. The big players across the medical-industrial complex joined the fight, threatened by limits to their profiteering. The disingenuously named Partnership for America's Health Care Future arose as a new alliance involving the hospital industry, the insurance industry, Big PhRMA, and for a time, physicians, with a multimillion campaign to defeat Medicare for All. They made all kinds of false assertions, such as: it would break the bank, it would be a socialist takeover of health care, people would lose benefits and choice, and wait times would go way up. [34, 35]

Conclusion:

The coronavirus pandemic shows how important it is to regulate our health care system. The U. S. was woefully unprepared and remained so well into the pandemic, when we became the world leader in terms of confirmed cases. The Trump administration failed to learn anything from experience abroad or in the early stages here. As a result, there was an ongoing dire shortage of critical life and death supplies, such as ventilators, N95 masks, and other protective gear for health care workers on the front lines of care. More people died than would have had our preparedness and management of this crisis been better.

The last 50 years in this country have demonstrated that market-based, laissez faire approaches to regulation in the public interest do not work. A larger role of responsive government is required. Theodore Roosevelt knew this in dealing with the Gilded Age of his times. His words are even more relevant today, more than a century later:

> *The great corporations... are the creatures of the State, and the State has not only the right to control them, but it is duty-bound to control them wherever the need for control is shown.*
>
> — President Theodore Roosevelt, 1902.

While this chapter has exposed the soft underbelly of system problems in U. S. health care, there are still more, especially in how we finance health care. We really do need to address these larger issues, including the questions of who is the health care system for, corporate profits vs. patients, and are we up to the challenge of reforming it in the public interest. We address them in the next and last chapter.

References:

1. Sparrow, MK. *License to Steal: How Fraud Bleeds America's Health Care System*. Boulder, CO. *Westview Press*, 2000, pp. 253-254.
2. Kuttner, R. *Everything for Sale: The Virtues and Limits of Markets*. Chicago, IL. *University of Chicago Press*, 1999, p. 140.
3. Greider, W. *Who Will Tell the People: The Betrayal of American Democracy*. New York. *Touchstone*, 1992, pp. 336-337.
4. Kuttner, R. Conservatives mugged by reality. *The American Prospect*, July/August, 2014: p. 5.
5. Ramsey, L, Friedman, L. The government agency in charge of approving drugs gets a surprising amount of money from the companies that make them. *Business Insider*, August 17, 2016.
6. Lupkin, S. Nearly 1 in 3 recent FDA approvals followed by major safety actions. *Kaiser Health News*, May 9, 2017.
7. Gaffney, A. Congress just quietly handed drug companies a dangerous victory. *New Republic*, December 14, 2016.
8. Prupis, N. Penalties for PhRMA crimes have all but disappeared, report finds. *Public Citizen News*, May/June 2018, p. 11.
9. Steinzor, R. The war on regulation. *The American Prospect*, Spring 2017, pp. 72-76.

10. Rowland, C, Johnson, CY, McGinley, L. Trump calls drug a 'game-changer,' but FDA says it needs further study. *The Washington Post*, March 20, 2020: A20.

11. Neuman, S. Man dies, woman hospitalized after taking form of chloroquine to prevent Covid-19. *NPR*, March 24, 2020.

12. Rowland, C. FDA approves use of unproven treatments, saying the risks are worthwhile. *The Washington Post*, March 31, 2020.

13. Lupkin, S. FDA grants experimental coronavirus drug benefits for rare disease treatments. *NPR*, March 24, 2020.

14. Demko, P. Healthcare's hired hands: When the stakes rise in Washington, healthcare interests seek well-connected lobbying firms. *Modern Healthcare*, October 6, 2014.

15. Ibid # 13.

16. Gilead must relinquish monopoly on potential coronavirus treatment. *Public Citizen*, March 25, 2020.

17. Thebault, R, Dupree, J, Hauslohner, A. U. S. death toll tops 100; experts expect rapid increase. *The Washington Post*, March 18, 2020: A 1.

18. Verma, S. As quoted by Drucker, J, Silver-Greenberg, J. Trump administration is relaxing oversight of nursing homes. *New York Times*, March 14, 2020.

19. Yong, E. How the pandemic will end. *The Atlantic*, March 25, 2020.

20. Lee, D, Haberhorn, J. Trump's refusal to use powers assailed. States are bidding against one another to get masks, ventilators. *Los Angeles Times*, March 26, 2020.

21. Sumner, M. Trump orders GM to make ventilators, without contract, at someone else's factory, by tweet. *Daily Kos*, March 27, 2020.

22. Johnson, J. Tracking tool shows fines for corporate misconduct plummeted under Trump. *Common Dreams,* February 13, 2018.

23. Claypool, R. Soft punishments lead to corporate law breaking. *Public Citizen News*, November/December, 2019, p. 6.

24. Saez, E, Zucman, G. *The Triumph of Injustice: How the Rich Dodge Taxes and How to Make Them Pay. W.W. Norton & Company.* New York, 2019: pp. vii-viii.

25. Phillips, AM, Christensen, K, Elmahrek, A. Stimulus benefits special interests: $2-trillion rescue plan includes long-sought boons for business. *Los Angeles Times*, March 27, 2020.

26. Altman, D. Surprise medical bills could be a powerful campaign issue. *Axios*, September 24, 2018.

27. Bluth, R, Huetteman, E. Investors' deep-pocketed push to defend surprise medical bills. *Kaiser Health News*, September 11, 2019.

28. Cunningham, PW. Congress is probing secretive groups opposing medical billing reforms. *The Washington Post*, September 17, 2019.

29. Mathews, AW. Hospitals to fight disclosure of prices. *Wall Street Journal*, November 21, 2019.

30. Armour, S. Hospital groups sue to keep rates secret. *The Washington Post*, December 5, 2019.

31. Huetteman, E, Hancock, J, Lucas, E. PhRMA cash rolls into Congress to defend an embattled industry. *Kaiser Health News*, August 27, 2019.
32. Tiku, N. Drug firms' Facebook ads spur privacy concerns. *The Washington Post*, March 6, 2020: A 1.
33. Feng, R. A new epidemic tests the limits of PhRMA's monopoly model. *Public Citizen News*, March/April 2020, p. 4.
34. Alonzo-Zaldivar, AP FACT CHECK: Trump distorts Democrats' health care ideas. *AP News*, October 9, 2018.
35. Cancryn, A. The army built to fight 'Medicare for All.' *Politico*, November 25, 2019.

Chapter 11

REFORM IS ACHIEVABLE,
BUT A MATTER OF POLITICAL WILL

*Rising health costs put health care reform on the agenda,
but the more likely a reform proposal is to control costs, the less
likely it is to be politically viable.* [1]

—Jonathan Oberlander, Ph.D., Professor of
Social Medicine at the University of North Carolina
and author of *The Political Life of Medicare*

*The U. S. and global economy do need a gigantic bailout
now to prevent suffering by innocent people resulting from both
the pandemic and economic collapse. But the bailout needs to
be focused, in the immediate, on delivering to everyone the
health care provisions that they need and to keeping people
financially whole. Taking a broader structural perspective,
we also need to stop squandering the enormous financial
privileges enjoyed by the U. S. on propping up the neoliberal
edifice that has dominated economic life in the U. S. and the
world for the past 40 years. . . . We could start by replacing
the private health insurance industry with Medicare for All. .
. . The U. S. economy that will emerge out of the present crisis
cannot be permitted to return to the neoliberal status quo.* [2]

—Robert Pollin, Professor of Economics at the University
of Massachusetts Amherst and founding co-director
of the Political Economy Research Institute

The first opening quote draws attention to a long-standing
barrier in U. S. politics over health care reform. Dr. Oberlander, who
has documented the history and evolution of Medicare so well over
the years, knows full well the power of money as the ultimate paradox

147

standing in the way of serious health care reform. The second quote brings us directly to the urgency of dealing with the coronavirus pandemic and the associated recession, if not depression.

Thank you, good reader, for hanging into this book to its last chapter. Here we have three goals: (1) to present the case for and against four alternatives for our health care system; (2) to discuss the battle royal ahead as these alternatives are debated by legislators, stakeholders and the public; and (3) to consider the road ahead, with or without real reform, during and after this crisis-packed election year.

But before we start, let's ask four essential questions to keep in mind as we go through these alternatives:

- Who is the health care system for—profiteering corporate stakeholders, their shareholders and Wall Street investors— or patients, families and taxpayers?
- Is health care just another commodity for sale in our largely for-profit market-based system—or essential services based on medical necessity?
- Is health care a human right or a privilege based on ability to pay?
- What ethic should prevail in health care—a business "ethic" maximizing revenue to providers or a service ethic based on needs of patients and their families?

I. Case For and Against Four Alternatives

Before reviewing our major options for health care reform, we need to start with where we are now.

1. The Status Quo, with Inadequate Response to the COVID-19 Pandemic

The case for the status quo is untenable. Instead, it requires drastic short- and long-term reform. Its failings are starkly exposed by the COVID-19 pandemic. We have had a delayed and poor response by the federal government—lack of planning; chronic underfunding of public health; no stockpiling of critical supplies and personal protective equipment; not enough testing kits, ventilators, hospital and ICU beds; and a shortage of physicians, nurses and other health professionals. According to *The New York Times*, the heads of major corporations and the U. S. Chamber of Commerce had lobbied the Trump administration against invoking the Defense Production Act in order to provide and distribute these essential supplies rapidly.[2] Trump has also shown a disdain for science, handing out false encouragement to the public without regard to the growing danger of the pandemic in this country and failing to set evidence-based national policy.

World-renowned philosopher Dr. Noam Chomsky, emeritus professor of linguistics at MIT and author of the 2016 book, *Who Rules the World?*, sums up our lack of preparedness this way:

> *The pandemic had been predicted long before its appearance, but actions to prepare for such a crisis were barred by the cruel imperatives of an economic order in which "there's no profit in preventing a future catastrophe."* [4]

A recent brief from Covered California, outlines the potential deleterious impacts that can be expected without decisive federal action, stating that "If these impacts are not mitigated, the public health and economic consequences to consumers, small and large employers and health insurers are potentially staggering, including:

- Consumers and employees not getting needed testing or treatments due to cost barriers, both for COVID-19 but also for other health conditions.
- Employers no longer being able to offer affordable coverage, or dramatically shifting costs to employees.
- Consumers and employers no longer being able to afford coverage, leading to employer groups dropping coverage or individuals deciding to go uninsured.
- Even more unsubsidized marketplace enrollees being priced out of individual markets.
- Small insurers risk insolvency, and if they close, put covered consumers at financial risk, damaging competition that benefits consumers and the employers that purchase on behalf of millions of Americans.
- Dramatic cost increases, many of which will be borne by the federal government in the form of higher Advanced Premium Tax Credits or by both federal and state governments paying for increased Medicaid enrollment as individuals and employers drop coverage." [5]

- The Trump administration, in refusing to serve as a national bargaining and distributional agent to deal with the COVID-19 pandemic, saying they were not a distributional agent and refusing to be a "shipping clerk," left states and cities bidding against each other and driving up prices. As a result, New York State had to pay 20 cents for gloves that normally cost less than 5 cents, and $2,795 for infusion pumps that normally cost less than one-half of that. [6]

These shortfalls are not surprising when we consider some comparisons with other advanced countries around the world.

- The U. S. has far fewer physicians and hospital beds than other countries, just 2.8 beds per 1,000 people compared to 13.1 and 12.3 in Japan and South Korea, respectively. [7]
- We rank last out of eleven advanced countries in terms of access to affordable care, quality of care, and outcomes. (Figure 11.1)
- We are the only country among these 11 not to have a solid system of universal coverage of health care.
- We spend far more than all of these other countries, get much less, including worse outcomes and more preventable deaths.
- Despite the ACA in 2010, there are still 30 million uninsured and 87 million underinsured Americans.
- We have a largely for-profit multi-payer health insurance system that sucks much of our health care dollar away from patient care through its high overhead, administrative costs and profits. Figure 11.2 compares U.S. health insurance overhead with five other countries.
- Almost one-third of total health spending goes to profiteering, waste, and fraud, as shown on p.126, and we have no reason to believe that these amounts are lower today.[8]

The status quo includes a massive, multi-payer private health insurance industry that profiteers in many ways on the backs of Americans in their vulnerabilities to becoming sick and/or disabled, as we saw in Chapters 5 and 6. It depends on employers to fund most of its coverage, but also receives $685 billion in federal subsidies each year, which the CBO expects to double in another ten years.[9] Despite all that, look at how private insurers have raised their

FIGURE 11.1

Overall Ranking of Eleven Health Care Systems

COUNTRY RANKINGS
Top 2*
Middle
Bottom 2*

	AUS	CAN	FRA	GER	NETH	NZ	NOR	SWE	SWIZ	UK	US
OVERALL RANKING (2013)	4	10	9	5	5	7	7	3	2	1	11
Quality Care	2	9	8	7	5	4	11	10	3	1	5
Effective Care	4	7	9	6	5	2	11	10	8	1	3
Safe Care	3	10	2	6	7	9	11	5	4	1	7
Coordinated Care	4	8	9	10	5	2	7	11	3	1	6
Patient-Centered Care	5	8	10	7	3	6	11	9	2	1	4
Access	8	9	11	2	4	7	6	4	2	1	9
Cost-Related Problem	9	5	10	4	8	6	3	1	7	1	11
Timeliness of Care	6	11	10	4	2	7	8	9	1	3	5
Efficiency	4	10	8	9	7	3	4	2	6	1	11
Equity	5	9	7	4	8	10	6	1	2	2	11
Healthy Lives	4	8	1	7	5	9	6	2	3	10	11
Health Expenditures/Capita, 2011	$3,800	$4,522	$4,118	$4,495	$5,099	$3,182	$5,669	$3,925	$5,643	$3,405	$8,508

Notes: *Includes ties, **Expenditures shown in $US PPP (Purchasing Power Parity). Australian $ data from 2010.

Source: Reprinted with permission from Davis, K, Stremikis, K, Squires, D et al. *Mirror, Mirror on the Wall, 2014 Update: How the U.S. Health Care System Compares Internationally.* The Commonwealth Fund, June 16, 2014.

FIGURE 11.2

INSURANCE OVERHEAD, UNITED STATES VS FIVE OTHER COUNTRIES, 2016

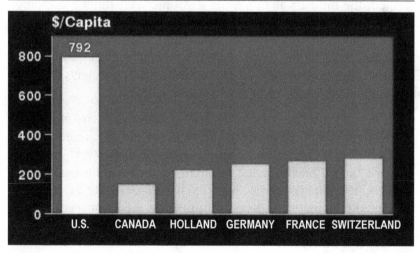

Source: OECD, 2016; NCHS; CIHI

prices over the last two years compared to those of hospitals and physicians.[10] (Figure 11.3)

FIGURE 11.3

HEALTH INSURANCE PRICES RISING FASTER, 2018-2020

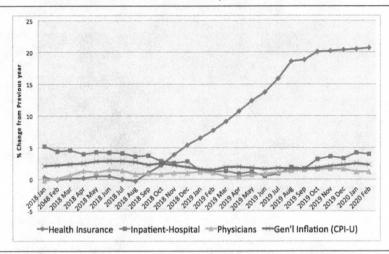

Source: U.S. Bureau of Labor Statistics

Since passage of the ACA in 2010, the industry has increased its role in privatizing managed care of public Medicare and Medicaid plans, with administrative overhead and profits of 18 to 20 percent compared to about 2.5 percent for traditional Medicare.[11] As expected, the industry is mounting a strong, well-funded campaign to defeat any plan for universal coverage through a public plan.

Opponents of single-payer Medicare for All warn us about the consequences of taking away employer-sponsored health insurance (ESI) that "covers" some 150 or 160 million Americans. But their pleas against such reform disregard these hard facts:

- Some 66 million Americans left or lost their jobs in 2018, with many not regaining health insurance in another job. ESI is further volatile, since the average American has had 12 jobs before reaching age 50, many not providing insurance benefits. When not employed, most have no health insurance.
- Benefits under ESI keep diminishing as employers limit benefits and as employees pay more in lost wages.
- General Motors decided to stop paying healthcare premiums for 49,000 striking workers in 2019. [12]

- As of April 1, 2020, four in ten Americans had lost their jobs or work-related income due to the coronavirus crisis, including more than one-half of part-time workers. [13]
- At that time, about 10 million Americans had filed for unemployment insurance, putting an unprecedented strain on Medicaid as a default insurance plan. [14] As we go to press, that number is more than 36 million people.

Wendell Potter was an executive with Cigna, later a senior fellow on health care at the Center for Media and Democracy, and is author of *Deadly Spin: An Insurance Company Insider Speaks Out on How Corporate PR Is Killing Health Care and Deceiving Americans*. After his long experience, he draws this conclusion about the effects of the coronavirus pandemic in this country:

> *The virus has caused a public health crisis so severe that people have been forced to stay home, causing businesses to shutter and lay off workers. And with roughly half of Americans getting their health insurance from their employer, these layoffs mean not only losing their income but also their medical coverage. In other words, just as our need for medical care skyrockets in the face of a global pandemic, fewer will have health insurance or be able to afford it.*
>
> *America needs to get out of the business linking health coverage to job status. Even in better times, this arrangement was a bad idea from a health perspective. Most Americans whose families depend on their employers for coverage are just a layoff away from being uninsured. And now, when many businesses are shutting down and considering layoffs, it's a public health disaster.* [15]

As Drs. Case and Deaton observe:

> *The historical accident of employer-based coverage is a huge barrier to reform. So is the way that the health care industry is protected in Washington by its lobbyists—five for every member of Congress. Our government is complicit in an extortion that is an important contributor to income inequality in America today. Through pharma companies that get rich by addicting people, and through excessive costs that lower wages and eliminate good jobs, the industry that is supposed to improve our health is undermining it.* [16]

2. Build on the Affordable Care Act (ACA)

Although some might think that building on the ACA might be easier politically, it is still under fire from the GOP, who have tried to kill it on several occasions. There is even a case still pending before the U. S. Supreme Court to determine whether it is constitutional. The GOP has still not come up with its own plan. But the case against it after 10 years is compelling.

While the ACA did bring improved access to health care to about 20 million people, mostly through expansion of Medicaid in 31 states, it has failed after ten years to rein in costs or sufficiently reform our system. Insurance and care remain unaffordable for much of our population. Private insurers have restricted access through narrow networks without adequate regulation; a Medicaid coverage gap was left in the 19 states refusing to expand Medicaid; and many insurers have abandoned markets that were not sufficiently profitable, often with little advance notice. [17] The ACA was never intended to achieve universal coverage, nor can it ever do so.

Dr. Don Berwick, former administrator of CMS, established in the early 2000s the Triple Aim as part of a National Quality Strategy—better care, healthier communities, and lower costs. Those goals have not been achieved. As he says today:

> *I see a loss of focus on quality and a loss of focus on universal coverage. In order to have quality healthcare, you have to have healthcare.* [18]

In a recent interview of presidential candidate Joe Biden by MSNBS's Yasmin Vossoughian, she asked this question: "Our health care system seems to be crumbling underneath this [COVID-19] crisis . . . Are you now reconsidering your position when it comes to single payer health care?" Biden responded: "Single payer will not solve all that." In response to that exchange, Dr. Don McCanne, family physician for some 35 years in Orange County, California and past president of Physicians for a National Health Program, had this rejoinder:

> *Sorry, Mr. Biden, you are wrong. All nations are now facing this pandemic. They each have to deal with the added costs of the burden placed on their public health systems and the costs of rendering health care to those who develop Covid-19. But the United States is unique in the instability in health care financing and coverage which will expose tens of millions to*

*personal financial hardship and possibly even bankruptcy.
That does not happen in nations that have stable, universal
health care financing systems.*

*Mr. Biden, a single-payer, Medicare for All program
would remove financial barriers to care and prevent financial
hardship due to medical bills. Yes, additional public health
measures are required, and the nation would benefit from
better social insurance programs covering other individual
and family costs related to the pandemic, but that is certainly
no reason to reject the vastly superior Medicare for All model
of financing health care. And remember, it is the people who
are the patients, not the commercial insurers.* [19]

In his dismissal of Medicare for All, Biden stated that Italy's
universal coverage system did not save them from so many
COVID-19 deaths in the pandemic. But that assertion exposed
his lack of understanding of Italy's health care system. Its original
national program has been decimated and "Americanized" over the
last ten-plus years by recurrent budget cuts, increasing privatization,
and reduced access to care similar to trends here in the U. S. [20]

3. Medicare for Some: Variants of a Public Option
Many moderate Democrats are touting the advantages of one or
another form of Medicare for Some, such as lowering the eligibility
age of Medicare, a Medicare buy-in for sale alongside private plans
on the ACA's exchanges; a pay or play plan, whereby employers
could choose between purchasing private insurance or paying a steep
payroll tax of about 8 percent; and a Medicare Advantage for All
plan, mimicking the private Medicare Advantage plan that so many
correctly label as Medicare Disadvantage, with all its disadvantages
described in previous chapters.

Democratic presidential candidate Joe Biden's middle-of-the-
road public option plan presumably builds on the ACA, thereby
leaving the private health insurance industry in place. It is weak on
details, but has these elements:

- Provides primary care without any copayments.
- Silent on other out-of-pocket costs.
- Would expand federal subsidies so that no one purchasing insurance on the individual market would pay more than 8.5 percent of their income on premiums.
- Would negotiate prices with providers.
- Would allow Medicare to negotiate drug prices, allow drug importation, and limit drug price increases to the rate of inflation using a tax penalty. [21]

While politically attractive to some, each variant of a public option has these kinds of problems: added administrative complexity and bureaucracy; restricted access to care; skimpy benefits; could never contain system-wide health care costs; would still leave many Americans uninsured, and could never achieve universal coverage; millions would still have high deductibles, as well as having little or no protection against surprise medical bills. Moreover, a public option would sacrifice about $350 billion a year of single payer's potential savings as well as another $220 billion a year in private insurers' overhead. [22]

4. Medicare for All

The case for Medicare for All is very strong. It is our only way out of the fix we find ourselves in. Our present corporatized market-based system lacks enough regulation to ensure access to health care of acceptable quality. Privatization of public programs, such as Medicare and Medicaid, has resulted in many abuses, including restricted access, higher costs, and worse care than their public counterparts. National polls have recorded a long descent in the public's trust and respect for corporations, with only Congress and HMOs lower. [23]

Expanded and Improved Medicare for All, as currently represented by H. R. 1384 bill in the House, when enacted, will bring:

- A new system of national health insurance (NHI), with equity for all U. S. residents, based on medical need, not ability to pay, and on the principle that health care is not a privilege but a human right.
- Universal access to health care for all U. S. residents, with full choice of providers and hospitals anywhere in the country without any restrictive networks.

- Coverage of all medically necessary care, outpatient and inpatient services; laboratory and diagnostic services; dental, hearing, and vision care; prescription drugs; reproductive health; maternity and newborn care; mental health services, including substance abuse treatment; and long-term care and supports.
- No cost-sharing such as copays and deductibles at the point of care; no more pre-authorizations or other restrictions now imposed by private insurers.
- Pharmaceutical reform, including negotiated drug prices.
- Administrative simplification with efficiencies and cost containment through large-scale cost controls, including (a) negotiated fee schedules for physicians and other health professionals, who will remain in private practice; (b) global budgeting of individual hospitals and other facilities; and (c) bulk purchasing of drugs and medical devices.
- Elimination of employer-sponsored health insurance and the private health insurance industry, with its onerous administrative overhead and profiteering.
- Allocation of 1 percent of its budget over the first five years for assistance and retraining of the estimated 1.7 million workers displaced by single-payer NHI.
- Cost savings that enable universal coverage through a not-for-profit single-payer financing system.
- Regional funding for rural and urban areas that are medically underserved.
- Improved quality of care and outcomes for both individuals and populations due to universal access to care and increased funding for public health.
- Shared risk for the costs of illness and accidents across our entire population of 326 million Americans. [24]

Single-payer Medicare for All will free physicians to focus on patient care, not wasteful billing and clerical activities that sap time and resources. It will establish a physician workforce plan with an emphasis on primary care and other shortage fields. It can save almost $600 billion in administrative waste from the current multi-payer financing system. [25] It can also reduce the poverty level by more than 20 percent by eliminating such out-of-pocket costs as deductibles, copays, coinsurance, and self-payments. [26]

As we have seen in earlier chapters, the private insurance industry has had a long run in this country, but has proven itself to have a mission of self-interest instead of the public interest. It was bailed out by the ACA with expanded markets and federal subsidies. But still today, ten years after enactment of the ACA, insurers still game the system at patients' expense through such means as higher cost-sharing, restrictive networks, deceptive marketing, and limited drug formularies. Its ongoing raison e'tre is to maximize revenue for CEOs and shareholders. But its many failings have now been further exposed as millions of workers lose their jobs across the country during and after the COVID-19 pandemic. [27]

It is long overdue to recognize the industry itself as a barrier to urgently needed reform. Such a change will be in concert with American values. (Table 11.1)

TABLE 11.1

Alternative Financing Systems and American Values

TRADITIONAL VALUE	Single-Payer	Multi-Payer
Efficiency	↑	↓
Choice	↑	↓
Affordability	↑	↓
Actuarial value	↑	↓
Fiscal responsibility	↑	↓
Equitable	↑	↓
Accountable	↑	↓
Integrity	↑	↓
Sustainable	↑	↓

Source: Geyman, JP. *Health Care Wars: How Market Ideology and Corporate Power Are Killing Americans.* Friday Harbor, WA. Copernicus Healthcare, 2012, p. 198.

Josh Bivens of the Economic Policy Institute sees Medicare for All as helping both the labor market and the economy. As he said some weeks into the coronavirus pandemic in the U. S.:

A national program that would guarantee health insurance for every American could:

- *Boost wages and salaries by allowing employers to redirect money they are spending on health care costs to their workers' wages.*
- *Increase job quality by ensuring that every job now comes bundled with a guarantee of health care—with the boost to job quality even greater among women workers, who are less likely to have employer-sponsored health care.*
- *Lessen the stress and economic shock of losing a job or moving between jobs by eliminating the loss of health care that now accompanies job losses and transitions.*
- *Support self-employment and small business development— which is currently super low in the U. S. relative to other rich countries—by eliminating the daunting loss of/cost of health care from startup costs.*
- *Inject new dynamism and adaptability into the overall economy by reducing "job lock'—with workers going where their skills and preferences best fit the job, not just to workplaces (usually large ones) that have affordable health plans.*
- *Produce a net increase in jobs as public spending boosts aggregate demand, with job losses in health insurance and billing administration being outweighed by job gains in provision of health care, including the expansion of long-term care.* [28]

An excellent study by the Political Economy Research Institute (PERI) at the University of Massachusetts Amherst found that single-payer Medicare for All will save the U. S. $5.1 trillion over a decade through savings from replacing our for-profit market-based, multi-payer financing system.

The PERI study set out this approach for progressive taxes:

1. Business premiums 8 percent below what a business now spends on health care.
2. 3.75 percent sales tax on non-essential goods.
3. Recurring tax of 0.36 percent on all wealth over $1 million.
4. Taxing long-term capital gains as taxable income.

Based on this approach, middle-class Americans will see savings of up to 14 percent, while high-income Americans will have only a small increase in their total health care spending. (Figure 11.4) [29]

FIGURE 11.4

Percent Change in Health Care Spending Under Medicare for All by Income Level and Insurance Status, 2016

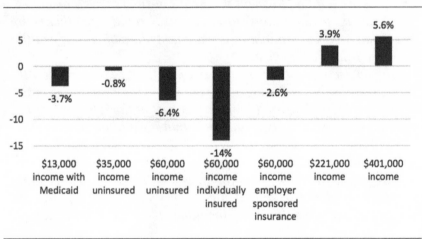

Sources: 2016 American Community Survey, the Consumer Expenditure Survey, and others.

Opponents of Medicare for All bring out their time-worn claims that it will restrict choice, ration care, cost too much, be less efficient than private health insurance, overrun our hospitals, and bring socialism. All these are belied by facts and long experience with traditional public Medicare. It has brought comprehensive benefits to its beneficiaries, with full choice of physician and hospital anywhere in the country, without rationing, and with a low administrative overhead of little more than 2 percent. As for potential hospital overrun, the hospitalization rate dropped from 12.8 per 100 Americans to 12.7 after its startup in 1965, while the numbers also dropped after the ACA in 2010, as patients could access earlier care. [30] Figure 11.5 illustrates the hypocrisy of opponents' fears of socialism.

FIGURE 11.5

IS SOCIAL SECURITY SOCIALISM?

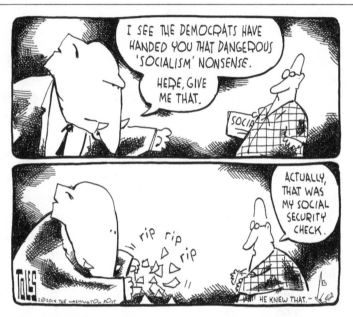

Sources: Permission from Tom Toles

The late Uwe Reinhardt, Ph.D., Professor of Political Economy, Economics and Public Affairs at Princeton University for almost 50 years, author of *Priced Out: The Economic and Ethical Costs of American Health Care*, and long a supporter in principle of Medicare for All, had this reservation about it in this country:

> *I have not advocated the single-payer model here because our government is too corrupt. Medicare is a large insurance company whose board of directors (Ways and Means and Senate Finance) accept payments from vendors to the company. In the private market, that would get you into trouble. . . . the key to a single-payer system is that the government sets prices. . . . The U. S. government is too corrupt to manage a single-payer system well.* [31]

Do we need to accept this conclusion, or can we demand competence, integrity and accountability through the democratic process this November?

II. A Battle Royal: Corporate Money and Wall Street vs. the American People

The proper role of government has long been a source of controversy, whether in the economy, health care or society. A larger role is strongly supported by progressives and many moderates, while conservatives on the right argue for a limited federal role with more governance at state and local levels.

Can we shed ourselves of the growing corporate bureaucracy, with all its profiteering and corruption, that takes health care away from our citizens with the false promises of choice and efficiency? So far, we can't, as Robert Reich, whom we met in Chapter 7, observes:

> *Corruption has become systemic, reaching deep into both political parties. While there are important differences between parties—Democratic members of Congress are far more socially liberal than Republicans and more concerned about poverty, climate, guns, and the rights of women and minorities—neither party is committed to challenging the increasing concentration of wealth and power in America. Both have come to depend on that wealth, and therefore defer to that power.* [32]

Returning to our task of deciding among our three reform alternatives going forward, Table 11.2 lays out the pros and cons of each.

So, given the best and only option that will ever bring universal coverage to the American people, what then should be the role of health-related corporations? Robert Reich, author of the 2020 book, *The System: Who Rigged It, How We Fix It*, wrote this to Jamie Dimon, Chair and CEO of JP Morgan Chase bank, the biggest and most influential bank in the country, and chairman of the Business Roundtable:

If you and the other members of the Business Roundtable were serious about becoming responsible to all your stakeholders, you'd use your formidable political power to reduce your power relative to them. You'd seek legislation binding yourself and every other major corporation to have worker representation on your boards of directors, mandating that workers receive a certain percentage of shares of stock, requiring that your corporations recognize a union when a majority of your workers want one, giving the communities where you operate a say before your corporations abandon them, and imposing higher corporate taxes in order to support your workers and your communities. [33]

Table 11.2

COMPARISON OF THREE ALTERNATIVES

	ACA	PUBLIC OPTION	MEDICARE for ALL
Access	Restricted	Restricted	Unrestricted
Choice	Restricted	Restricted	Unrestricted
Cost containment	Never	Never	Yes
Quality of care	Unacceptable	Unacceptable	Improved
Bureaucracy	Increased	Increased	Much reduced
Universal coverage	Never	Never	Yes, immediately
Accountability	No	No	Yes
Sustainability	No	No	Yes

As the political debate plays out during this election season and beyond, we can only hope that Big Money, Big Corporations, and the likes of Jamie Dimon, with all their spending, don't win the day against the public good. The huge lobbying effort to defeat

Medicare for All, together with members in the top 1 % and 10% in both chambers of Congress, are potential barriers to real reform (Figure 11.6).

FIGURE 11.6

FINANCIAL WEALTH DISTRIBUTION IN THE U.S. HOUSE AND SENATE

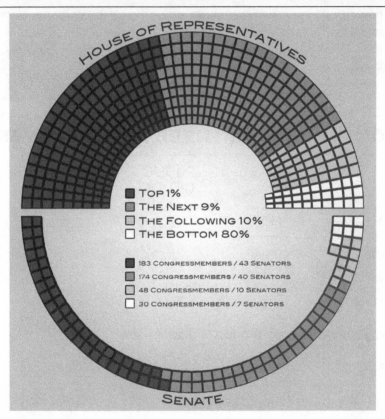

Source: University of California, Santa Cruz, UCSC.edu, sociology, Who Rules America, Power, Wealth

Of the 100 members of the Senate, 93 are in the top 10 percent of wealth in our country; of the 435 members of the House of Representatives, 405 are also in that category. They are elected to represent us all, but can they understand and empathize with the stresses that ordinary Americans contend with, especially during and after this pandemic and recession/depression?

III. The Road Ahead—With or Without Real Reform

This is where we are now in our present predicament in the U.S., hopefully not the "new normal," in the grip of the COVID-19 pandemic with its uncertain future around the world:

- Ranks of uninsured estimated by an economist at the Federal Reserve Bank to surge to 47 million by the end of June, 2020; more than 7 million newly uninsured by then. [34]
- Not enough physicians, nurses and other health care professionals.
- Lack of a national physician workforce plan, especially for shortage fields in primary care, geriatrics and psychiatry.
- Not enough hospital beds; some hospitals, especially in rural areas, threatened by closure. [35]
- Underfunded and under-appreciated public health.
- Too much waste, especially through an exploitive private insurance industry.
- Increasing inequality and health care disparities.
- Too many Americans dying early, preventable deaths.
- Plenty of money in our system, just needing to be redirected to the public interest, not more profits to a corporatized marketplace and Wall Street investors.
- Federal stimulus/support packages being debated in Congress so far not earmarking funds for coverage of COVID-19 treatment.
- Growing opposition to financing reform that would threaten corporate profits and move health care to a more service-oriented ethic.

I am sorry that Bernie Sanders is not the Democratic Party's final presidential candidate in the 2020 elections, but as Robert Reich has so well said:

> *The country is far better off because of your unrelenting courage and commitment to the progressive change we so desperately need in a country so riddled with inequality and division. Four years ago, in the 2016 Democratic primaries, you made it respectable to talk about Medicare for All, free public higher education, and raising taxes on the wealthy. You alerted America to the vast and growing gap in income, wealth, and political power, and its dangers for our economy and democracy.* [36]

165

Medicare for All is all the more important now as a crucial approach to address the nation's crisis with the COVID-19 pandemic, made worse by the Trump administration's delayed and ineffective response. Figure 11.7 shows how far behind the U. S. is compared to the other hardest hit countries. [37]

FIGURE 11.7

CONFIRMED COVID-19 CASES, DEATHS, AND RECOVERIES BY COUNTRY

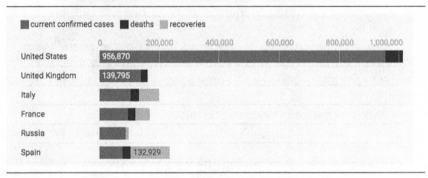

Source: Johns Hopkins, CSSEGISandData/COVID-19/datawrapper

As a long-time leader toward Medicare for All and lead sponsor of the Senate's bill, S-1129, Senator Bernie Sanders continues his dedication to this goal in these words, after passing the torch to the front-running Democratic presidential candidate, Joe Biden:

Today, families all across the country face financial hardship unimaginable only a few months ago. And because of the unacceptable levels of income and wealth distribution in our economy, many of our friends and neighbors have little or no savings and are desperately trying to pay their rent or their mortgage or even to put food on the table. This reality makes it clear to me that Congress must address this unprecedented crisis in an unprecedented way that protects the health and economic wellbeing of the working families of our country, not just powerful special interests. As a member of the Democratic leadership in the United States Senate, and as a senator from Vermont, this is something that I intend to be intensely involved in, and which will require an enormous amount of work. [38]

This important insight shines a bright light on the barriers that for so long have blocked universal coverage for all Americans:

> *The real struggle for a universal single payer system in the U. S. is not technical or economic but almost entirely political. Retaining anything resembling the status quo is the least disruptive and therefore politically easiest, route. Unfortunately, it is also the least effective route to attack the underlying pathology of the American healthcare system—corporatism run amok. Adopting the easiest route will do little more than kick the can down the road and will require repeatedly revisiting the deficiencies in our healthcare system until we get it right.* [39]

—Peter Arno, Ph.D., Health Policy Research Political Economy Research Institute, University of Massachusetts, Amherst and Philip Caper, M. D., internist with long experience in health policy since the 1970s and past chairman of the National Council on Health Planning and Development

One example of corporate stakeholders trying to take advantage of the COVID-19 pandemic is lobbyist backed H. R. 6514, the Worker Health Coverage and Protection Act (note the deceptive wording!), whereby the federal government would temporarily take responsibility for COBRA premium payments. Health insurers are already pocketing increased revenues due to widespread cancellation of elective procedures, then the federal government once again bails them out on the backs of workers, who still have to pay deductibles, co-insurance, co-pays, and out-of-network bills. Three former White House economists have correctly described this bill as "corporate welfare."

Fortunately, two other emergency bills are expected to be debated in Congress this summer. The Medicare Crisis Program Act (Jayapal/Kennedy) would enroll laid off workers in Medicare and cover all costs of COVID-related treatment. The Health Care Emergency Guarantee Act (Jayapal/Sanders) would enroll ALL uninsured U. S. residents in Medicare for the duration of the pandemic. Either bill would be much better for patients and their families than the corporate friendly H. R. 6514. [40]

As this debate continues through to and beyond the 2020 elections, we need real information on the pros and cons of these alternatives to reform our system. Instead, we are seeing a blizzard of disinformation and even outright lies that cloud the debate.

One major example of that is what Medicare for All will cost. The best studies, as discussed in this chapter, show that 95 percent of Americans will pay less that they do now for insurance and health care while getting universal coverage. At the same time, the federal government (and us taxpayers!) will save the $685 billion that we are paying each year to subsidize a failing private health insurance industry. [41] Other lies put forward by the opposition are that there will be rationing and long waiting lines. But look at where we are now—rationing by ability to pay and not gaining access to care!

Conclusion:

We have a political teeter totter in play. On one end are corporate money, Wall Street traders and investors, and those many profiteers in our free-wheeling market-based system. On the other end are physicians, nurses and other health professionals committed to serving the public without fiscal and bureaucratic barriers between them and their patients. They are buoyed by the latest Politico/ Harvard poll that finds that more than three-quarters of Republicans and Democrats rank "taking steps to lower the cost of health care" as "extremely" or "very" important—the top priority of Americans.[42]

This is a critical juncture to the future of American health care. Can we "drain the swamp" from corruption that has accelerated under the Trump administration, despite his original "promise?" Can we increase funding and the central role of public health at all levels—federal, state and county? And can we understand the extent of fundamental restructuring of health care that gets to the common good and away from profiteering against the public interest? Are we up to these challenges, or do we end up with dithering and more failed incremental "reforms" that miss the mark?

The answer to how we deal with these challenges will test our democracy to the core. Given the stakes, we'd better be up to coping with them, since they will make all the difference for generations to come.

For what lies ahead, we can take heart and support from these words by President Franklin Delano Roosevelt in his second inaugural address on January 20, 1937:

> *The test of our progress is not whether we add more to the abundance of those who have so much; it is whether we provide enough for those who have too little.*

References:

1. Oberlander, J. The politics of health care reform: Why do bad things happen to good plans? *Health Affairs Web Exclusive*, August 27, 2003.
2. Pollin, R. As interviewed by Polychroniou, CJ. Chomsky and Pollin: To heal from COVID-19, we much must imagine a different world. *Truthout*, April 10, 2020.
3. Chamber of Commerce lobbying against use of Defense Production Act. *Corporate Crime Reporter* 34 (13): p. 7, March 30, 2020.
4. Chomsky, N. As quoted by Polychroniou, CJ. Chomsky: Ventilator shortage exposes the cruelty of neoliberal capitalism. *Truthout*, April 1, 2020.
5. The Potential National Health Cost Impacts to Consumers, Employers and Insurers Due to the Coronavirus Covid-19). *Covered California*, March 22, 2020.
6. Reich, R. But the real hoax is Trump's committment to America. *Inequality Media*, April 5, 2020
7. Altman, D. Why the U. S. doesn't have more hospital beds. *Axios*, March 30, 2020.
8. Best Care at Lower Cost. Washington, D.C. Institute of Medicine, 2013, Table 3.1.
9. Ockerman, E. It costs $685 billion a year to subsidize U. S. health insurance. *Bloomberg News*, May 23, 2018.
10. Arno, PS, Caper, P. Medicare for each of us in the age of the coronavirus. *Common Dreams*, April 3, 2020.
11. Potter, W. Take it from me, tweaks won't fix health care. Democrats should focus on Medicare for All. *USA Today*, December 14, 2018.
12. Johnson, J. Progressives say GM's decision to cut off employee health insurance 'yet another reason why we need Medicare for All. *Common Dreams*, September 18, 2019.
13. Poll: 4 in 10 Americans report losing their jobs or work-related income due to the coronavirus crisis, including more than one-half of part-time workers. *Kaiser Family Foundation*, April 2, 2020.
14. Luthra, S, Galewitz, P, Bluth, R. Medicaid nearing 'eye of the storm' as newly unemployed look for coverage. *Kaiser Health News*, April 3, 2020.
15. Potter, W. Millions of Americans are about to lose their health insurance in a pandemic. *The Guardian*, March 27, 2020.
16. Case, A, Deaton, A. The sickness of our system. *Time*, March 2-9, 2020, p. 81.
17. Adelberg, M, Bagley, N. Struggling to stabilize: 3Rs litigation and the future of the ACA exchanges. Health Affairs Blog, August 1, 2016.

18. Berwick, D. as quoted by Castellucci, M. An opportunity lost with the National Quality Strategy. *Modern Healthcare*, March 23, 2020.
19. McCanne, D. Quote of the Day, Fate of commercial insurance under the COVID-19 Pandemic. Response to MSNBC's Yasmin Vossoughian, Y. on April 6, 2020.
20. Disamistade, V. No, Italy is Not the Case Against Medicare for All. *The Nation*, April 14, 2020.
21. Cohrs, R. Medicare for All vs. public option. *Modern Healthcare*, March 9, 2020, p. 12.
22. Himmelstein, DU, Woolhandler, S. The 'public option' on health care is a poison pill. *The Nation*, October 21, 2019.
23. Pearlstein, S. When shareholder capitalism comes to town. *The American Prospect*, March/April 2014: 40-48.
24. Geyman, JP. *Common Sense: The Case For and Against Medicare for All. Leading Issue in the 2020 Elections*. Friday Harbor, WA. *Copernicus Healthcare*, 2019, pp. 3-4, 22.
25. Gaffney, A, Woolhandler, S, Angell, M et al. Moving forward from the Affordable Care Act to a Single-Payer System. *Am. J Public Health* 106 (6): 987-988, 2016.
26. Bruenig, M. Medicare for All would cut poverty by over 20 percent. People's Policy Project, September 12, 2019.
27. Conley, J. 'We need Medicare for All': Massive coronavirus job losses expose obvious failure of employer-based insurance. *Common Dreams*, March 26, 2020.
28. Bivens, J. Fundamental health reform like 'Medicare for All' would help the labor market. *Economic Policy Institute*, March 5, 2020.
29. Higginbotham, T. Medicare for All is even better than you thought. Jacobin, December 3, 2018.
30. Gaffney, A. Can we afford Medicare for All? *The Boston Globe,* July 23, 2019.
31. Reinhardt, UE. *Priced Out: The Economic and Ethical Costs of American Health Care*. Princeton, NJ. *Princeton University Press*, 2019, p. 153.
32. Reich, RB. *The System: Who Rigged It, How We Fix It*. New York. *Alfred A. Knopf. Penguin Random House*, 2020, p. 69.
33. Ibid # 32, pp. 194-195.
34. Woolhandler, S, Himmelstein, DU. Intersecting U. S. epidemics: COVID-19 and lack of health insurance. *Annals Intern Med*, April 7, 2020.
35. Weber, L. Coronavirus threatens the lives of rural hospitals already stretched to breaking point. *Kaiser Health News*, March 22, 2020.
36. Reich, R. Letter to Bernie Sanders, April 8, 2020
37. Leonhardt, D. Not winning this fight. *New York Times*, March 31, 2020.
38. Sanders, B. The campaign ends, the struggle continues. April 8, 2020.
39. Arno, P, Caper, P. American health care—The illusion of choice. *Physicians for a National Health Program*, March 25, 2020.
40. Personal communication, Drs. Phil Caper and Peter Shapiro, May 6, 2020
41. Ibid # 9.
42. McDonough, JE. Medicare for All: What history can teach us about its chances. *Health Affairs Blog*, February 24, 2020.

Index

A

B

N

O

P

Q

R

reform, 165
Reich, Robert, 165-167
Reinhardt, author of Priced Out, 161–162 (quote)
Republicans against women's health care, 94–95
Rizvi, Zain, 143 (quote)
Riverside Medical Group, example, 122
Roe v. Wade Supreme Court decision on abortion, 94
Roosevelt, Theodore, President, 144 (quote)
Rosenthal, Dr. Elizabeth, 36, 103 (quote), 118–19
    (quote re husband's bill))
Rothman, Joshua, 89
rural health care and aging population, 96

S

Saez, Emmanuel, 127
Saini, Dr. Vikas, 48 (quote)
Salama, Rasha, 70
Salerno, Alexander, 122 (in quote)
Sanders, Bernie, 165, 166
Sanofi prices for insulin, 71
Scheide, Walter, 131 (quote)
Schierer-Radcliff, Jesima, insulin death, 71
Scully, Tom, 10 (quote)
seniors, high costs of health care, 73
Shankaran, Dr. Veena, 57 (quote)
shingles vaccine, insufficient, 108
Shkreli, Martin, guilty CEO, 108
SmithKline Beecham Clinical Laboratories, false billings, 2
socialism, fears, 161 (Fig. 11.5)
Spain, Barcelona-based Grifols family fraud, 112
Sparrow, Malcolm (License to Steal)
    British Police Service, 1
    License to Steal book, 1, 23–24, 71–72 (quote), 113, 133
Stark, Pete, 13–14 (quote)
Starr, Paul, Pulitzer Prize winning book, 8
Stiglitz, Joseph, 81 (quote)
Stoller, Matt, writer and budget analyst, 2–3, 8, 30, 103–104
    (quotes)

ABOUT THE AUTHOR

John Geyman, M.D. is professor
emeritus of family medicine at the
University of Washington School of
Medicine in Seattle, where he served as
Chairman of the Department of Family
Medicine from 1976 to 1990. As a
family physician with over 21 years in
academic medicine, he also practiced
in rural communities for 13 years. He
was the founding editor of *The Journal
of Family Practice* (1973 to 1990) and

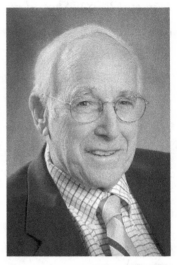

the editor of *The Journal of the American Board of Family Medicine*
from 1990 to 2003. Since 1990 he has been involved with research
and writing on health policy and health care reform.

His most recent book was *Long Term Care in America - The
Crisis All of Us Will Face in Our Lifetimes.* Earlier books include:
*TrumpCare: Lies, Broken Promises, How It Is Failing, and What
Should Be Done?* (2018), *Crisis in U.S. Health Care: Corporate
Power vs. the Common Good* (2017), *The Human Face of
ObamaCare: Promises vs. Reality and What Comes Next* (2016),
*How Obamacare Is Unsustainable: Why We Need a Single-Payer
Solution For All Americans* (2015), *Health Care Wars: How Market
Ideology and Corporate Power Are Killing Americans* (2012),
Souls On a Walk: An Enduring Love Story Unbroken by Alzheimer's
(2012), *Breaking Point: How the Primary Care Crisis Threatens*

the Lives of Americans (2011), *Hijacked: The Road to Single Payer in the Aftermath of Stolen Health Care Reform* (2010), *The Cancer Generation: Baby Boomers Facing a Perfect Storm* (2009), *Do Not Resuscitate: Why the Health Insurance Industry Is Dying* (2008), *The Corrosion of Medicine: Can the Profession Reclaim Its Moral Legacy* (2008), *Shredding the Social Contract: The Privatization of Medicare* (2006), *Falling Through the Safety Net: Americans Without Health Insurance* (2005), *The Corporate Transformation of Health Care: Can the Public Interest Still Be Served?* (2004), *Health Care in America: Can Our Ailing System Be Healed?* (2002), and *The Modern Family Doctor and Changing Medical Practice* (1971).

John has also published three pamphlets following the approach of Thomas Paine in 1775-1776: *Common Sense About Health Care Reform in America* (2017), *Common Sense: U.S. Health Care at a Crossroads in the 2018 Congress* (2018), and *Common Sense: The Case For and Against Medicare For All. Leading Issue in the 2020 Elections* (2019).

He also served as the president of Physicians for a National Health Program from 2005 to 2007, and is a member of the National Academy of Medicine.

CPSIA information can be obtained
at www.ICGtesting.com
Printed in the USA
BVHW081629210721
612419BV00004B/135